Tendon Reconstruction and Transfers of the Foot and Ankle

Editor

CHRISTOPHER L. REEVES

CLINICS IN PODIATRIC MEDICINE AND SURGERY

www.podiatric.theclinics.com

Consulting Editor
THOMAS ZGONIS

January 2016 • Volume 33 • Number 1

ELSEVIER

1600 John F. Kennedy Boulevard • Suite 1800 • Philadelphia, Pennsylvania, 19103-2899

http://www.theclinics.com

CLINICS IN PODIATRIC MEDICINE AND SURGERY Volume 33, Number 1
January 2016 ISSN 0891-8422, ISBN-13: 978-0-323-41466-1

Editor: Jennifer Flynn-Briggs
Developmental Editor: Alison Swety

Clinics in Podiatric Medicine and Surgery (ISSN 0891-8422) is published quarterly by Elsevier Inc., 360 Park Avenue South, New York, NY 10010-1710. Months of issue are January, April, July, and October. Business and Editorial Offices: 1600 John F. Kennedy Blvd., Ste. 1800, Philadelphia, PA 19103-2899. Customer Service Office: 3251 Riverport Lane, Maryland Heights, MO 63043. Periodicals postage paid at New York, NY and additional mailing offices. Subscription prices are $285.00 per year for US individuals, $498.00 per year for US institutions, $100.00 per year for US students and residents, $370.00 per year for Canadian individuals, $602.00 for Canadian institutions, $435.00 for international individuals, $602.00 per year for international institutions and $220.00 per year for Canadian and foreign students/residents. To receive student/resident rate, orders must be accompanied by name of affiliated institution, date of term, and the *signature* of program/residency coordinator on institution letterhead. Orders will be billed at individual rate until proof of status is received. Foreign air speed delivery is included in all *Clinics* subscription prices. All prices are subject to change without notice. POSTMASTER: Send address changes to *Clinics in Podiatric Medicine and Surgery*, Elsevier Health Sciences Division, Subscription Customer Service, 3251 Riverport Lane, Maryland Heights, MO 63043. **Customer Service: 1-800-654-2452 (US). From outside of the US, call 314-447-8871. Fax: 314-447-8029. E-mail: JournalsCustomerService-usa@elsevier.com (for print support); JournalsOnlineSupport-usa@elsevier.com (for online support).**

Reprints. For copies of 100 or more of articles in this publication, please contact the Commercial Reprints Department, Elsevier Inc., 360 Park Avenue South, New York, NY 10010-1710. Tel.: 212-633-3874; Fax: 212-633-3820; E-mail: reprints@elsevier.com.

Clinics in Podiatric Medicine and Surgery is covered in *MEDLINE/PubMed (Index Medicus) and EMBASE/Excerpta Medica.*

CLINICS IN PODIATRIC MEDICINE AND SURGERY

CONSULTING EDITOR
THOMAS ZGONIS, DPM, FACFAS

Contributors

CONSULTING EDITOR

THOMAS ZGONIS, DPM, FACFAS
Professor and Fellowship Director, Division of Podiatric Medicine and Surgery, Department of Orthopaedic Surgery, University of Texas Health Science Center at San Antonio, San Antonio, Texas

EDITOR

CHRISTOPHER L. REEVES, DPM, MS, FACFAS
Orlando Foot and Ankle Clinic, Winter Park, Florida; Attending Physician, Department of Podiatric Surgery, Florida Hospital East Orlando Surgical Residency Program, Orlando, Florida

AUTHORS

ERIC A. BARP, DPM, FACFAS
Foot and Ankle Surgeon, The Iowa Clinic, West Des Moines; Residency Director, Unity Point Health, Des Moines, Iowa

STEPHEN A. BRIGIDO, DPM, FACFAS
Department Chair and Fellowship Director, Foot and Ankle Department, Foot and Ankle Reconstruction, Coordinated Health, Bethlehem, Pennsylvania

MICHELLE BUTTERWORTH, DPM, FACFAS
Private Practice, Pee Dee Foot Center, Kingstree, South Carolina

JORDAN D. CAMERON, DPM
Podiatric Medicine and Surgery Resident (PGY-2), Florida Hospital East Orlando Residency Training Program, Orlando, Florida

ALAN R. CATANZARITI, DPM, FACFAS
Director of Residency Training Program, Division of Foot and Ankle Surgery, West Penn Hospital, Allegheny Health Network, Pittsburgh, Pennsylvania

RICHARD DERNER, DPM, FACFAS
President, American College of Foot and Ankle Surgeons; Private Practice, Associated Foot and Ankle Centers of Northern Virginia, Lake Ridge, Virginia; Member, Residency Training Committee, Inova Fairfax Medical Campus, Falls Church, Virginia

ANDREW D. ELLIOTT, DPM, JD
Podiatric Medicine and Surgery Resident (PGY-III), Gundersen Medical Foundation, La Crosse, Wisconsin

JOHN G. ERICKSON, DPM
Resident Physician, Unity Point Health, Des Moines, Iowa

CAITLIN S. GARWOOD, DPM, AACFAS
Diabetic Limb Salvage Fellow, Department of Plastic Surgery, Center for Wound Healing and Hyperbaric Medicine, MedStar Georgetown University Hospital, Washington, DC

BRIAN P. GRADISEK, DPM, AACFAS
Fellow, Weil Foot and Ankle Institute, Des Plaines, Illinois

SEAN T. GRAMBART, DPM, FACFAS
Orthopedics, Carle Physician Group, Champaign, Illinois

MATTHEW HENTGES, DPM
Foot and Ankle Surgery, West Penn Hospital, Pittsburgh, Pennsylvania

JEFFREY HOLMES, DPM
Podiatric Residency, Inova Fairfax Medical Campus, Falls Church, Virginia

MICHAEL A. HOWELL, DPM
Surgical Resident, Division of Foot and Ankle Surgery, West Penn Hospital, Allegheny Health Network, Pittsburgh, Pennsylvania

JAMES T. MASKILL, DPM
Orthopaedic Associates of Kalamazoo, Portage, Michigan

JENNIFER L. MULHERN, DPM, AACFAS
Fellow, Foot and Ankle Department, Foot and Ankle Reconstruction, Coordinated Health, Bethlehem, Pennsylvania

TREVOR PAYNE, DPM
Podiatric Surgical Resident (PGY-2), Florida Hospital East Orlando Residency Training Program, Orlando, Florida

GREGORY C. POMEROY, MD
New England Foot and Ankle Specialist and Director; Associate Clinical Professor, University of New England, Portland, Maine

NICOLE M. PROTZMAN, MS
Research Associate, Clinical Education and Research Department, Coordinated Health, Allentown, Pennsylvania

CRYSTAL L. RAMANUJAM, DPM, MSc
Assistant Professor/Clinical, Division of Podiatric Medicine and Surgery, Department of Orthopaedics, University of Texas Health Science Center at San Antonio, San Antonio, Texas

CHRISTOPHER L. REEVES, DPM, MS, FACFAS
Orlando Foot and Ankle Clinic, Winter Park, Florida; Attending Physician, Department of Podiatric Surgery, Florida Hospital East Orlando Surgical Residency Program, Orlando, Florida

THOMAS S. ROUKIS, DPM, PhD, FACFAS
Attending Staff, Departments of Orthopaedics, Podiatry, and Sports Medicine, Gundersen Health System, La Crosse, Wisconsin

AMBER M. SHANE, DPM, FACFAS
Orlando Foot and Ankle Clinic, Orlando, Florida; Attending Physician, Department of Podiatric Surgery, Florida Hospital East Orlando Surgical Residency Program, Orlando, Florida

DEVIN C. SIMONSON, DPM, AACFAS
Attending Staff, Departments of Orthopaedics, Podiatry, and Sports Medicine,
Gundersen Health System, La Crosse, Wisconsin

JOHN J. STAPLETON, DPM, FACFAS
Associate, Foot and Ankle Surgery, VSAS Orthopaedics, Chief of Podiatric Surgery,
Lehigh Valley Hospital, Allentown, Pennsylvania; Clinical Assistant Professor of Surgery,
Penn State College of Medicine, Hershey, Pennsylvania

JOHN S. STEINBERG, DPM, FACFAS
Professor, Department of Plastic Surgery; Co-Director, Center for Wound Healing and
Hyperbaric Medicine, MedStar Georgetown University Hospital, Georgetown University
School of Medicine; Program Director, Podiatric Residency Program, MedStar
Washington Hospital Center, Washington, DC

RYAN VAZALES, DPM
Podiatric Medicine and Surgery Resident (PGY-1), Florida Hospital East Orlando
Residency Training Program, Orlando, Florida

MATTHEW F. VILLANI, DPM
Chief, Podiatric Surgical Resident (PGY-3), Florida Hospital East Orlando Residency
Training Program, Orlando, Florida

LAURA WALTON, DPM
Private Practice, Daytona Beach, Florida

LOWELL WEIL Jr, DPM, MBA, FACFAS
Weil Foot and Ankle Institute, Des Plaines, Illinois

FRANCESCA ZAPPASODI, DPM
Chief, Podiatric Surgical Resident (PGY-3), Florida Hospital East Orlando Residency
Training Program, Orlando, Florida

THOMAS ZGONIS, DPM, FACFAS
Professor and Fellowship Director, Division of Podiatric Medicine and Surgery,
Department of Orthopaedic Surgery, University of Texas Health Science Center at San
Antonio, San Antonio, Texas

Contents

Foreword: Tendon Reconstruction and Transfers of the Foot and Ankle   xv

Thomas Zgonis

Preface: A New Look at Tendon Transfers and Soft Tissue Management in Foot and Ankle Reconstruction   xvii

Christopher L. Reeves

Principles and Biomechanical Considerations of Tendon Transfers   1

Laura Walton and Matthew F. Villani

> Whether performed as a primary procedure or used to augment and support osseous reconstruction, tendon transfers are a key skill for the foot and ankle surgeon. Understanding the biomechanics preoperatively and postoperatively is essential in performing appropriate procedures and in supporting patients throughout the rehabilitation process. Often the complexity of tendon transfer surgery is lost because it is deemed a soft tissue procedure and in theory should be less complex than osseous procedures. However, the dynamic nature of musculature and tendons require a deeper understanding of surgical and biomechanical concepts.

Flexor Digitorum Longus Tendon Transfer and Modified Kidner Technique in Posterior Tibial Tendon Dysfunction   15

James T. Maskill and Gregory C. Pomeroy

> The modified Kidner procedure and flexor digitorum longus tendon transfer are common procedures used today when addressing posterior tibial tendon dysfunction. These techniques are often used in conjunction with a combination of osteotomies to correct flatfoot deformity, and have been proved to be reliable and predictable.

Tibialis Anterior Tendon Transfer for Posterior Tibial Tendon Insufficiency   21

Crystal L. Ramanujam, John J. Stapleton, and Thomas Zgonis

> The Cobb procedure is useful for addressing stage 2 posterior tibial tendon dysfunction and is often accompanied by a medial displacement calcaneal osteotomy and/or lateral column lengthening. The Cobb procedure can also be combined with selected medial column arthrodesis and realignment osteotomies along with equinus correction when indicated.

Posterior Tibial Tendon Transfer   29

Amber M. Shane, Christopher L. Reeves, Jordan D. Cameron, and Ryan Vazales

> When performed correctly with the right patient population, a tibialis posterior muscle/tendon transfer is an effective procedure. Many different methods have been established for fixating the tendon, each of which has its own indications. Passing through the interosseous membrane is the

preferred and recommended method and should be used unless this is not possible. Good surgical planning based on patient needs and expectations, along with excellent postoperative care including early range of motion and physical therapy, minimizes risk of complications and allows for the optimal outcome to be achieved.

Tibialis Anterior Tendon Transfer   41

Jennifer L. Mulhern, Nicole M. Protzman, and Stephen A. Brigido

Tendon transfer procedures are used commonly for the correction of soft tissue imbalances and instabilities. The complete transfer and the split transfer of the tibialis anterior tendon are well-accepted methods for the treatment of idiopathic equinovarus deformity in children and adults. Throughout the literature, complete and split transfers have been shown to yield significant improvements in ankle and foot range of motion and muscle function. At present, there is insufficient evidence to recommend one procedure over the other, although the split procedure has been advocated for consistently achieving inversion to eversion muscle balance without overcorrection.

Jones Tendon Transfer   55

Richard Derner and Jeffrey Holmes

Hallux malleus is a deformity of the great toe. There is a dorsiflexion contracture at the metatarsophalangeal joint and plantar flexion of the interphalangeal joint. The deformity is commonly attributed to muscular imbalances of the various structures acting on the great toe. Jones tendon transfer is a procedure used to remove the deforming force to the clawed hallux. It is most often performed in conjunction with a hallux interphalangeal joint fusion. Typically there is a neurologic component causing a deformity to the entire foot, necessitating adjunct procedures. The Jones tendon transfer has shown to have reproducible results.

Hibbs Tenosuspension   63

Sean T. Grambart

Hibbs tenosuspension is an underutilized procedure when it comes to dealing with lesser toe pathology in conditions such as Charcot-Marie-Tooth disease. This article describes the procedure to transfer the extensor digitorum longus tendons into the peroneus tertius tendon to eliminate a deforming force and create a stabilizing force.

Tendon Transfers for Management of Digital and Lesser Metatarsophalangeal Joint Deformities   71

Michelle Butterworth

 Video of Flexor Tendon Transfer for 2nd MTPJ instability accompanies this article

Managing digital and metatarsophalangeal joint (MTPJ) deformities can range from simple to complex and uniplanar to triplanar. Because of the complexity and variability of digital and MTPJ deformities, there are many procedures, and no one procedure has become the gold standard.

Tendon transfers for digital and MTPJ deformities are just one treatment option, and usually they are not stand-alone procedures. Typically, a combination of procedures needs to be performed. This article describes the surgical technique and provides a review of the literature, including clinical results for tendon transfers of the central rays.

Tendon Transfers and Salvaging Options for Hallux Varus Deformities   85

Brian P. Gradisek and Lowell Weil Jr

Hallux varus is an infrequently encountered deformity of the first ray characterized by a medial deviation of the hallux on the first metatarsal head at the first metatarsal phalangeal joint. Iatrogenic flexible hallux varus often requires surgical repair to create a functional, pain-free, shoeable foot. Although arthrodesis remains the mainstay of treatment, many soft tissue transfer procedures have been described in the literature as joint-sparing alternatives to fusion. This article explores in detail the tendon transfer procedures that have been described for repair of flexible hallux varus deformity.

Soft Tissue Balancing After Partial Foot Amputations   99

Caitlin S. Garwood and John S. Steinberg

Partial foot amputations have become common procedures for the foot and ankle surgeon as part of a limb salvage practice. These procedures are highly technique driven and there are many complex factors that affect the outcome and longevity. Appropriate surgical planning must be used with every partial foot amputation to ensure a plantigrade foot with the least potential for future breakdown. When performed appropriately, these amputations have great success with lower energy expenditure and decreased mortality compared with below-knee or above-knee amputations.

Flexor Hallucis Longus Tendon Transfer for Calcific Insertional Achilles Tendinopathy   113

Michael A. Howell and Alan R. Catanzariti

 Video of surgical technique for the treatment of CIAT with FHL tendon transfer accompanies this article

Calcific insertional Achilles tendinopathy can result in significant pain and disability. Although some patients respond to nonoperative therapy, many patients are at risk for long-term morbidity and unpredictable clinical outcomes. There is no evidence-based data to support the timing of operative invention, choice of procedures, or whether equinus requires treatment. This article suggests the need for a classification system based on physical examination and imaging to help guide treatment. There is an obvious need for evidence-based studies evaluating outcomes and for properly conducted scientific research to establish appropriate treatment protocols.

Combined Tendon and Bone Allograft Transplantation for Chronic Achilles Tendon Ruptures   125

Alan R. Catanzariti and Matthew Hentges

Combined flexor hallucis longus tendon transfer and bone-tendon allograft transplantation is a reasonable option for advanced distal-segment

Achilles tendinopathy. This procedure provides anatomic restoration and improved function of the posterior muscle group without sacrificing the regional anatomy. Allograft transplantation is safe and does not require immunosuppressive therapy. The soft tissue envelope should be healthy because wound complications can be an issue. This procedure is especially helpful in patients with significant disability.

Surgical Correction of Rigid Equinovarus Contracture Utilizing Extensive Soft Tissue Release   **139**

Christopher L. Reeves, Amber M. Shane, Francesca Zappasodi, and Trevor Payne

Although deforming contractures of the lower extremities after acute cerebrovascular events are well documented in the literature, there is limited literature regarding specific surgical considerations for the correction of these deformities, which are nonosseus in nature. The equinovarus foot, regardless of its origin, is a challenging pathologic condition for the foot and ankle surgeon. It is critical to have a firm understanding of the cause and symptoms behind an equinovarus deformity before treatment. The clinical presentation is discussed with special attention to deformities in adults with rigid equinovarus deformities after cerebrovascular-related accidents or peripheral ischemic events.

Catastrophic Failure of an Infected Achilles Tendon Rupture Repair Managed with Combined Flexor Hallucis Longus and Peroneus Brevis Tendon Transfer   **153**

Devin C. Simonson, Andrew D. Elliott, and Thomas S. Roukis

Deep infection is one of the most devastating complications following repair of an Achilles tendon rupture. Treatment requires not only culture-driven antibiotic therapy but, more importantly, appropriate débridement of some or even all of the Achilles tendon. This may necessitate delayed reconstruction of the Achilles tendon. The authors present a successful case of reconstruction of a chronically infected Achilles tendon in an otherwise healthy 43-year-old man via a multistaged approach using the flexor hallucis longus and peroneus brevis tendons. We also provide a brief review of the literature regarding local tendon transfer used in the reconstruction of Achilles tendon rupture.

Complications of Tendon Surgery in the Foot and Ankle   **163**

Eric A. Barp and John G. Erickson

This article discusses four subsets of patients that have an increased risk of complications from tendon surgery in the foot and ankle: smokers, diabetics, and patients with peroneal or Achilles tendon pathology. Very little has been published on the complications of other tendon surgeries in the foot and ankle other than Achilles tendon repair. Data can be extrapolated from the general orthopedic literature and animal studies to help guide therapy and treatment options. The foot and ankle surgeon must take into account the entirety of the history and physical examination to develop a treatment plan that optimizes each patient's chance for a complication-free recovery.

Index   **177**

CLINICS IN PODIATRIC MEDICINE AND SURGERY

FORTHCOMING ISSUES

April 2016
Nerve-Related Injuries and Treatments for the Lower Extremity
Stephen L. Barrett, *Editor*

July 2016
Dermatological Manifestations of the Lower Extremity
Tracey C. Vlahovic, *Editor*

October 2016
Current Update on Foot and Ankle Arthroscopy
Sean T. Grambart, *Editor*

RECENT ISSUES

October 2015
Secondary Procedures in Total Ankle Replacement
Thomas S. Roukis, *Editor*

July 2015
Foot and Ankle Osteotomies
Christopher F. Hyer, *Editor*

April 2015
Sports Related Foot & Ankle Injuries
Paul R. Langer, *Editor*

January 2015
Current Update on Orthobiologics in Foot and Ankle Surgery
Barry I. Rosenblum, *Editor*

RELATED INTEREST

Clinics in Sports Medicine, October 2015 (Vol. 34, Issue 4)
Sports Injuries in the Foot and Ankle
Anish R. Kadakia, *Editor*
Available at: http://www.sportsmed.theclinics.com/

Raphael L. Barrett, Editor

Foreword

Tendon Reconstruction and Transfers of the Foot and Ankle

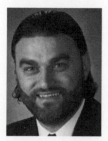

Thomas Zgonis, DPM, FACFAS
Consulting Editor

This issue of *Clinics in Podiatric Medicine and Surgery* is dedicated to tendon reconstruction and transfers of the foot and ankle, including and not limited to tendon transfers for toe deformities, posterior tibial tendon dysfunction, Achilles tendon ruptures, and equinovarus deformities. Equal attention is placed on the principles and biomechanics of tendon transfers as well as soft tissue balancing procedures for diabetic partial foot amputations. Last, complications of tendon surgery in the foot and ankle are also discussed in detail.

Tendon surgery in the foot and ankle is very common and may be combined with osseous reconstructive procedures when necessary. In this issue, the guest editor, Dr Christopher L. Reeves, along with the invited authors, has done a superb job in addressing some of the most common tendinous reconstructive procedures performed in the foot and ankle. I would like to thank all of our readers and authors again for their continuous support and outstanding submissions.

Thomas Zgonis, DPM, FACFAS
Division of Podiatric Medicine and Surgery
Department of Orthopaedic Surgery
University of Texas Health Science
Center at San Antonio
7703 Floyd Curl Drive-MSC 7776
San Antonio, TX 78229, USA

E-mail address:
zgonis@uthscsa.edu

Clin Podiatr Med Surg 33 (2016) xv
http://dx.doi.org/10.1016/j.cpm.2015.10.002
0891-8422/16/$ – see front matter © 2016 Published by Elsevier Inc.

Preface

A New Look at Tendon Transfers and Soft Tissue Management in Foot and Ankle Reconstruction

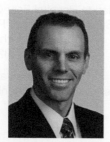

Christopher L. Reeves, DPM, MS, FACFAS
Editor

When presenting the topic of tendon repair and reconstruction of the lower extremity, it is commonplace to immediately focus on the Achilles tendon. While the majority of the research and surgical techniques are centered on the Achilles tendon, this issue of *Clinics in Podiatric Medicine and Surgery* moves outside of the box and focuses not only on tendon reconstruction but also on the mechanical redistribution of tendon function.

Since the late 19th century, surgeons have been modifying the function of tendons (lengthening, transfers, transpositions, and so on) to restore anatomy and function to a disabled extremity. While early procedures were employed primarily in treating neuromuscular disorders, today we know that tendon transfer surgery is a mainstay in reconstructive foot and ankle surgery, including flatfoot and posttraumatic disorders, to name a few.

We have recruited some of the best-known surgeons in foot and ankle surgery as well as a few rising stars of our profession to present you with an all-encompassing issue of tendon transfer management, soft tissue deformity reconstruction, and complication management. I would like to commend our authors on their work and offer my sincere gratitude on their tremendous time and effort that they put forth in preparing their articles. In addition, I would like to thank Dr Thomas Zgonis and the staff at Elsevier for their guidance in developing this issue.

Tendon transfers and tendon reconstruction has become one of my personal favorite surgeries to perform. I have found the results to be dramatic and predictable, and the patient population undergoing the procedure to be one of the most appreciative of the results. I hope that you enjoy reading these articles as much as I have. In addition, it

Clin Podiatr Med Surg 33 (2016) xvii–xviii
http://dx.doi.org/10.1016/j.cpm.2015.10.001
0891-8422/16/$ – see front matter © 2016 Published by Elsevier Inc.

podiatric.theclinics.com

is hoped that the guidance and pearls provided here will offer you significant clinical guidance in the decision-making and positive outcomes for your patients.

Christopher L. Reeves, DPM, MS, FACFAS
Orlando Foot and Ankle Clinic
2111 Glenwood Drive, Suite 104
Winter Park, FL 32792, USA

Department of Podiatric Surgery
Florida Hospital East Orlando
Surgical Residency Program
7727 Lake Underhill Road
Orlando, FL 32828, USA

E-mail address:
creeves@orlandofootandankle.com

Principles and Biomechanical Considerations of Tendon Transfers

Laura Walton, DPM[a], Matthew F. Villani, DPM[b],*

KEYWORDS

- Tendon transfers • Biomechanics of tendon transfers • Anatomy of the tendon
- Principles of tendon transfers • Tendon surgery

KEY POINTS

- Although there is no guarantee for a perfect tendon transfer, the guarantee of failure increases exponentially if a surgeon is not following the principles of tendon transfers.
- When determining the appropriate tendon for transfer, the surgeon must evaluate multiple different properties of the muscle and tendon.
- Tendon transfers can provide large amounts of correction whether used alone or concomitantly with other procedures.

INTRODUCTION

The majority of the literature on tendon transfers is with respect to the upper extremity, but the principles and biomechanics of tendon transfers often are interchangeable and can be used in foot and ankle procedures as well. The outbreak of pollo in the nineteenth century was the marked onset of the utilization of tendon transfers in the lower extremity to improve patients' ambulatory status. The first tendon transfer in the foot and ankle was in 1881, with an attempt to replace a paralyzed triceps surae with the peroneal tendons.[1,2]

TENDON ANATOMY

To understand the subtle complexities of tendon transfers and biomechanics, what makes a tendon unique must first be understood. The histology and biological makeup

No commercial or financial conflicts of interest and no funding source for this article.
[a] Private Practice, 1890 LPGA Boulevard, Suite 230, Daytona Beach, FL 32117, USA; [b] Florida Hospital East Orlando Residency Training Program, 7727 Lake Underhill Road, Orlando, FL 32828, USA
* Corresponding author.
E-mail address: villanidpm@gmail.com

of the tendon make it a different subject matter from bone and it requires different care to garner desired results. Understanding the limits and capabilities of individual tendons allows surgeons to push the envelope and develop new techniques. Hand surgeons, along with the maxillofacial surgeons, foot and ankle surgeons, and orthopedic surgeons, have been the modern-day pioneers of tendon transfer surgery. Different surgeries may have different goals, but often in tendon transfer surgery, balance is more important than shear strength.[2] Not only is a full understanding of the individual tendon being transferred needed, but also an understanding functional requirements of the limb. Tendons are unique entities that play many roles within the functionality of the body. Tendons function to transfer load from muscle to bone throughout their complex composition and hierarchal structure.[3]

Histology

The structure of the tendon is a straightforward hierarchy. Small collagen fibers link together into a linear chain. These linear chains then link together to form fibrils. These fibrils are bundled together to form fascicles, which are covered in a layer of endotenon. Lastly, there is an epitenon, which encapsulates the entire tendon and a layer of fluid before being covered by the paratenon (**Fig. 1**). The paratenon and endotenon supply blood to the midsubstance of the tendon. In cases of tendons without a paratenon, the central tendon blood supply is via the vinicula (or plica) within the tendon sheath. In its natural form, tendon is composed predominantly (approximately 70% by dry weight) of type I collagen with small amounts of proteoglycan's, glycoprotein, and minor collagens.[4]

Tendons are relatively avascular, consisting of 30% collagen, 2% elastin, and 68% water. A decrease in collagen weakens the tendon (discussed later). Collagen formation is also a vital determining factor for postoperative rehabilitation. Inactivity can result in increased collagen degradation, decreased tensile strength, and decreased concentration of metabolic enzymes.[5] Despite adequate and healthy collagen levels, tendons can still tear if pushed beyond their capabilities. The strength of the tendon is often described using a stress-strain curve or Blix curve (discussed later).

Blood Supply

The blood supply of the tendon is highly variable and is usually divided into 3 regions: (1) the musculotendinous junction, (2) the midsubstance of tendon, and

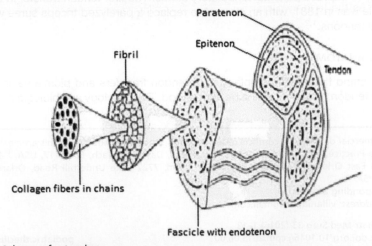

Paratenon

Epitenon

Fibril

Tendon

Collagen fibers in chains

Fascicle with endotenon

Fig. 1. Makeup of a tendon.

(3) the tendon bone junction[5] (**Fig. 2**). The amount of vascularity can vary from tendon to tendon and is most often compromised in the Achilles tendon, tibialis posterior tendon, and supraspinatus tendon. These tendons are left particularly vulnerable to injury and difficulties with healing. The tibialis posterior tendon has a rich supply of blood at its musculotendinous and osseous junctions, but there is an area of hypovascularity posterior and distal to the medial malleolus.[6] The Achilles tendon is one of the strongest in the body, but its fascicles also have one of the highest degrees of twisting, which produces stress, notably at 2 to 5 cm proximal to the insertion. This is also the area of the lowest vascularity and highest chance of injury.[5] In these areas of low vascularity, it is believed that synovial and lymphatic fluids supply some nourishment. Blood supply is important for injury prevention, healing, production collagen, and minimizing adhesions. Preserving the blood supply during tendon transfers increases the odds of a successful transfer with desired long-term outcomes.

Innervation

The nerve supply of the tendon is largely, if not exclusively, afferent. The afferent receptors are the Golgi tendon organs (GTOs) found at the neuromuscular junction.[5] There is also some research to show that a small portion of innervation is from independent deep and superficial nerve fibers. GTOs control muscle tension because they respond to tension rather than length and adjust accordingly. An increase in muscle tension causes a proportionate increase in discharge frequency of a GTO. When the nerve supply to the tendon becomes compromised, that GTO loses its ability to regulate the tendon contractures. Without that regulation, the muscle, and even the limb, can become spastic or flaccid. Refer to **Box 1** for a list of nerve disorders that commonly lead to tendon dysfunction. Some of these diseases are more amenable to tendon transfer surgery than others. Iatrogenic nerve damage affecting the tendon is rare, but it is one of the many reasons why an extensive knowledge of anatomy is crucial prior to performing any operation. The ability of a tendon to contract and stretch is the key to its strength.[5]

Tendon Strength

When the tendon is relaxed, the collagen fibers are in a relaxed wavy overlapping pattern. As the tendon is pulled straight, the collagen fibers straighten as well. At a

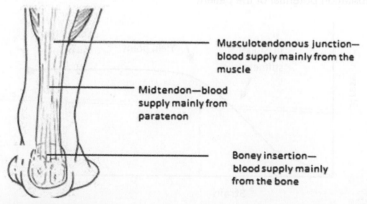

Musculotendonous junction—blood supply mainly from the muscle

Midtendon—blood supply mainly from paratenon

Boney insertion—blood supply mainly from the bone

Fig. 2. Blood supply to tendon.

> **Box 1**
> **Nerve disorders commonly leading to tendon dysfunction**
>
> - Poliomyelitis
> - Charcot-Marie-Tooth disease
> - Multiple sclerosis
> - Discogenetic disease (with nerve impingement)
> - Sciatic nerve palsy
> - Common peroneal nerve palsy (leading to drop foot)
> - Ankylosing spondylitis

certain point of stretch, the collagen fails and the tendon ruptures. This can be determined using the stress-strain curve (**Fig. 3**). Physiologic loading is less than 4% stress, which is a safe zone; past 8% stretch, the tendon ruptures.[7] The capacity at which a tendon can tear can be affected by outside factors, such as age and health of the host. This is because the outside factors can directly of indirectly affect the amount of collagen present.

The length-tension curve (Blix curve) further examines the strength (tension a muscle can endure) in relationship to the amount it is stretched (sarcomere length) (**Fig. 4**). Although the relationship of tension to sarcomere length is set, the sarcomere length has the ability to adapt. The myofilaments within a sarcomere can increase or decrease their overlap depending on the demands they incur. This becomes a crucial concept in determining the insertion point for tendon transfers. When the tendon is inserted at or slightly beyond its rest length, it is at its maximal tension. If the insertion point is too proximal or too distal, the strength is decreased. The resting length represents the position from which the muscle can generate its greatest force and it is reflected by the muscle fiber length, which depends on the sarcomere length.[8–11]

PATIENT EVALUATION

As with any surgical procedure, preoperative planning is imperative with tendon transfers. To have a successful outcome requires a team approach with the surgeon, patient, and physical therapist. Preoperatively, assessment is important to determine the rehabilitation potential of the patient.

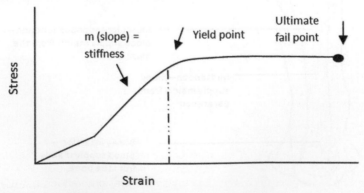

Fig. 3. Stress-strain curve.

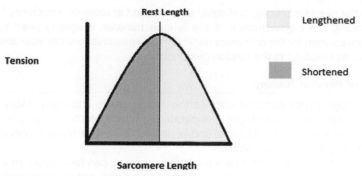

Fig. 4. Blix curve.

First, evaluating individual patients is important to differentiate between the different pathologies resulting in their dysfunction. Each patient has different functional needs, expectations, and limitations that need to be determined and discussed preoperatively. Some common disorders that result in deformities that could benefit from tendon transfers are neuromuscular disorders, peripheral nerve injuries, central nervous system injuries, and trauma resulting in loss of muscle or tendon function. Determining if a pathology is progressive or nonprogressive is imperative. Both upper and lower motor neuron lesions can result in a progressive deformity. Upper motor neuron lesions secondary to central nervous system pathology most commonly result in spastic or progressive disorders. Lower motor neuron lesions typically result in paralysis or flaccid muscle tone.[12,13]

Patient Selection

A patient's other comorbidities have to be taken into account prior to surgery. The ideal patient is rare, and it is the burden of the surgeon to determine which risks are acceptable and which patients are suitable candidates. Patients with multiple comorbid conditions, such as diabetes, require tendon transfers and many have been shown to effect soft tissue composition. Connizzo and colleagues[3] investigated the mechanical properties of muscles and tendons of mice with diabetes and demonstrated that tendons were smaller in diameter and transition strain occurred significantly earlier in the stress-strain curve in the diabetic mice than in the control group.

Alterations in collagen structure have been seen with increasing age and diabetes. In aging patients, type I collagen becomes less flexible and more acid insoluble, leading to the accumulation of advanced glycation end products. The effect of advanced glycation end products on tendons results in alteration in protein interaction with the matrix and between cells, which leads to reduced healing capacity and altered mechanical properties of connective tissue.[14] The presence of glycation end products is a normal part of aging; however, research is showing similar amounts of glycation end products in younger diabetic patients. These patients generally have less flexibility in their tendons and are at an increased risk for injury.[3]

Patient Goals

Surgeons must understand patients' functional needs and be able to explain to patients that they may not return to preinjury level even with a successful outcome. The goal of the tendon transfer is not to replace the previous tendon but to redirect the pull and better balance the foot, eliminate deforming forces, correct deformity, eliminate the need for braces, and delay deterioration of osseous structures.[1,2] Before understanding the biomechanics of the tendon transfer, surgeons need to have a strong appreciation for the pathomechanics of the causative foot disorder and the disease process resulting in the tendon dysfunction.

The Role of Physical Therapy

Obtaining appropriate consults prior to the procedure is important. Many patients need to be seen by a neurologist preoperatively, where electromyography or nerve conduction studies can be ordered and reviewed. Having a patient evaluated by a physical therapist is also beneficial.[2,15]

The preoperative physical therapy evaluation not only can help establish a relationship, which can be beneficial in the postoperative course, but also can give the therapist the ability to develop a treatment plan and obtain preoperative measurements and functionality scores. The reduction of joint contractures and increase of range of motion of the affected and ancillary joints preoperatively can help to optimize outcomes postoperatively. Having an open trusting relationship with the therapist is essential and, when choosing a therapist, the surgeon must insure that the therapist is aware of what the surgical procedure entails and the limitations a patient might have postoperatively.[2]

Preoperative Muscle Evaluation

When determining the appropriate muscle/tendon for transfer, the surgeon must evaluate multiple different properties of the muscle and tendon. The tendon must be of adequate strength to perform the new function. Grading of muscle strength from 0 to 5 has been described, ranging from full strength against resistance to no contraction (**Box 2**). During the tendon transfer, the muscle loses 1 muscle grade; therefore, the recommendation of only transferring tendons with a muscle grade of 4 or 5 has been made. The surgeon must determine, however, if the tendon transfer to function is expected in a static or dynamic manner. Tendons with a lower muscle grade can be used if performing a static function is ideal.[16] The specific properties of the muscle also should be taken into account.

The overall strength of a muscle is its capacity to generate tension. When determining the force of a muscle, it is found proportional to the physiologic cross-sectional area of the muscle belly.[16–18] Muscle excursion is the muscle length necessary to produce the full joint ROM. This can be influenced by the moment arm, which is the distance the insertion is from the joint axis of rotation; therefore, the larger the moment arm the smaller the excursion and vice versa.[17,19] This concept is discussed later. Silver and colleagues[17] performed a cadaver study to compare the work capacity of the

---

Box 2
Muscle grade

Grade 0: No contraction

Grade 1: Visible/palpable contraction but no movement

Grade 2: Movement with gravity eliminated

Grade 3: Movement against gravity only

Grade 4: Movement against gravity with minimal resistance

Grade 5: Movement against gravity with full resistance

different muscles in the lower extremity. They removed all other soft tissue, leaving only muscle belly. They took the total weight of all harvested muscles and determined a percentage for each individual muscle, allowing them to calculate a work capacity for each (**Table 1**). The soleus was found to have the highest work capacity and strength, and the extensor hallucis longus had the largest excursion. Muscles with similar strength percentage have similar force-generating capacities; muscles with similar fiber lengths have similar excursion potential.

As discussed previously, balancing of the foot is important but this is not an absolute when dealing with the antagonist tendons of the feet. The plantar flexors account for 54.5% of the force in the foot, but the dorsiflexors account for only 9.4% of the force. In the theory of balance, they should be equal, but a different amount of strength is necessary for these muscle groups to perform their function. The primary function of the dorsiflexors is not propulsion but to clear the ground during swing phase; therefore, a larger force is needed from the plantar flexors.[17] This is an example of why knowing the functionality of the tendons and the anatomy of the entire body unit is important.

RULES OF TENDON TRANSFERS

Although there is no guarantee for a perfect tendon transfer, the guarantee of failure increases exponentially if a surgeon is not following the principles of tendon transfers. These principles have been studied and expanded on for generations. No 1 rule is more important than another; they work in unison to insure the best result. The 7 rules of tendon transfers are discussed and **Box 3** lists them.

The Absence of Fixed Deformity

Full passive ROM of all involved joints is needed for a successful active transfer. If a joint is stiff or immobile, a new tendon is not able to overcome the deformity. When a mild contracture is present, conservative methods of correction are preferred

Table 1 Strength percentages of muscles in the lower leg	
Muscle	**Strength Percentage**
Soleus	29.9
Medial head of gastrocnemius	13.7
Tibialis posterior	6.4
Tibialis anterior	5.6
Lateral head of gastrocnemius	5.5
Peroneus longus	5.5
Flexor hallucis longus	3.6
Peroneus brevis	2.6
Flexor digitorum longus	1.8
Extensor digitorum longus	1.7
Extensor hallucis longus	1.2
Peroneus tertius	0.9
Plantaris	0.7

Data from Silver RL, de la Garza J, Rang M. The myth of muscle balance. A study of relative strengths and excursions of normal muscles about the foot and ankle. J Bone Joint Surg Br 1985;67(3):432–7.

Box 3
Principles of tendon transfers

1. The absence of fixed deformities
2. Suitable soft tissue bed
3. Selection of donor tendon with similar strength and excursion
4. Expendable donor
5. Straight line of pull
6. Synergy
7. Single function per transfer
---

because surgical intervention can lead to scarring and potentially increased contractures and should be reserved for moderate to severe contractures and osseous deformities. Conservative treatment is accomplished most commonly with aggressive physical therapy or serial casting.[13,19]

The forces required of a new tendon transfer to a supple joint are far less than the forces required to move a stiff or contracted joint due to increased drag and resistance.[20] In severe or long-standing cases of decreased joint mobility, the objective is improvement rather than perfection. This is often achieved with surgeries, such as joint capsule release, arthroscopic débridement, exostectomy, and so forth. If contracture release is necessary, it should be performed before the transfer procedure and followed by intensive therapy to ROM.[13] This cannot be accomplished if the contracture release is performed simultaneously with the tendon transfer because the tendon needs a period of immobilization to heal at its attachment point. Most osseous procedures can be performed, however, at the same time as a tendon transfer because they either benefit from or be unaffected by the immobilization period (eg, exostectomy and correctional osteotomies). In foot surgery, tendons often cross more than 1 joint; each joint should be assessed and addressed individually.

Suitable Soft Tissue Bed

The soft tissues surrounding a newly transferred tendon should ideally be undamaged. The tissue bed should be free of edema, inflammation, and scar to allow for unrestricted tendon movement. If unable to avoid an area of undesirable tissue, it should be addressed prior to or during the surgical transfer. Minimizing adhesions as a part of tendon transfers is addressed preoperatively, intraoperatively, and postoperatively.[13,16,19]

Selection of Donor Tendon with Similar Strength and Excursion

Excursion is the linear movement of a tendon needed to perform a desired action. The strength of the tendon is its ability to withstand forces; a muscle's cross-sectional area can determine this. The cross-sectional area of a muscle compared with another muscle is, therefore, a measure of relative strength of the muscles.[17] Because relative strength is a constant, some investigators have hypothesized that this is more valuable to know than the absolute strength when choosing the tendon for transfer. If a tendon is too strong or does not have enough excursion, it can potentially cause negative outcomes. The average strength and excursion of an individual muscle and tendon within the lower extremity are different from those of the hand and upper extremity. Average values have been studied and chronicled, notably by Silver and colleagues.[17] These values serve only as a guide; patients should be assessed on an individual basis (discussed previously).

Expendable Donor

The principle of using an expendable muscle-tendon unit as a donor means that there must be another remaining muscle that continues to adequately perform the transferred muscle-tendon unit's original function. There is some redundancy of tendons in the foot (multiple flexors and extensors), which allows for harvest of these tendons with minimal effects on function. With smaller joints there is also the option of joint arthrodesis. The benefits of the harvest must outweigh the decrease in function afforded by the joint arthrodesis.[13,19]

Straight Line of Pull

For the most optimal function, surgeons want the line of pull of the transferred tendon to be parallel with the recipient muscle and in a straight line from the origin to insertion. Although this is preferable, it is not always practical secondary to the location of the origin compared with the new insertion. This might require routing a structure around an osseous structure or through an interosseous membrane. Any divergent angle of pull can result in decreased strength and function; it can also be used as an advantage because the angle of pull can help further correct the deformity.[2,8,13,19]

Synergy

Although each muscle has a specific function, muscle groups work together to perform a desired function. During the preoperative evaluation and planning, using muscles for the transfer that normally function together can help produce a more favorable outcome. Synergistic transfers are favorable but not always practical, depending on the disease processes resulting in the muscular deficiency in the first place. Nonsynergistic transfers often require more postoperative rehabilitation to get the tendon to function in phase. If there is failure at this phase, the tendon may function only in a static state. This aspect of synergy is also referred to as in-phase or out-of-phase transfers in the foot in and ankle, referring to muscles that function in the swing phase or stance phase of gait.[13,19] The swing phase muscles consist of the tibialis anterior, extensor hallucis longus, extensor digitorum longus, and peroneus tertius. The tibialis posterior, flexor digitorum and hallucis longus, gastrocnemius, soleus, and peroneus brevis and longus are all stance phase muscles. With in-phase transfers, function of the tendon has been demonstrated in 7 to 8 weeks. In certain incidences, phase conversion is not as important as functional conversion, where the tendon can be trained to perform a desired function with rehabilitation.[7]

Single Function per Transfer

When choosing a tendon to be transferred, surgeons should look at the primary deficit and attempt to correct that deformity. The tendon transfer should be responsible for the restoration of 1 lost function. When an attempt is made to have the tendon transfer correct multiple defects and have multiple functions, the strength and movement from the primary concern are compromised. If the tendon transfer passes multiple joint axis, however, it could result in multiplanar correction.[13,19]

INTRAOPERATIVE CONSIDERATIONS TO IMPROVE OUTCOMES

Within the confines of the operating room, there are small considerations that can increase the chance of desirable outcomes. These range from appropriate handling of tissues to different surgical techniques. There are some techniques that are highly debatable, such as the use of synthetic graft, whereas others are more agreed on. Minimally invasive and no-touch techniques are widely accepted as the standard when performing tendon transfers. Although the use of these techniques cannot guarantee an improved outcome, they are considered standard of care and should be used whenever possible. All techniques are meant to improve the quality of the transfer by decreasing trauma to the tendon and reducing the risk of adhesions.[16] There are certain tips and tricks used to improve specific tendon transfers, discussed elsewhere in this issue.

Reduction of Adhesions

With any tendon transfer, some degree of adhesion is going to develop. Limiting the adhesions is beneficial and can be the difference between a favorable and poor outcome. Surgeons must pay attention to the soft tissue envelope that the tendon transfer is going to course through (discussed previously). During surgery, no-touch techniques (using K wires for retraction, skin hooks with minimal tension, and so forth) are ideal. The less tension on the subcutaneous tissues, the less likely they are to develop thick scars. Limit the exposure of the tendon to the outside environment, keep the tendon moist, and do not wrap tendon in moist gauze because the gauze can be abrasive and cause trauma to the tendon or paratenon. When handling the tendon, do so at the distal aspect, this area is used for fixation or resected after the transfer is complete most commonly.[1,16,21]

Transfers should either be performed open, to avoid tension on small incisions, or through minimally invasive tunnels. To create the tunnels, a small incision is made at the musculotendinous junction of the harvest tendon, at the insertion of the harvest tendon, and at the site of transfer. The tendon is then released and rerouted through a series of small incisions with the use of a soft tissue tunneling devices. The device is blunt and there is minimal chance for neurovascular damage. The subcutaneous and subcuticular tissue is left untouched and ideally does not scar. This technique is best used with long transfers from the leg to the foot and is more difficult to perform with short transfers from the ankle.[4,16]

When at all possible, preserve the paratenon to prevent adhesion and maintain blood supply. Voleti and colleagues[4] found that after injury, tendons can heal via intrinsic proliferation and migration of tenocytes from the epitenon and endotenon or by extrinsic factors with invasion of cells from the surrounding sheath and synovium. Intrinsic proliferation is preferable and prevents adhesions. When the synovial sheath is damaged, it allows granulation tissue and tenocytes to invade the repaired area. When this happens, the exogenous cells outnumber the endogenous tenocytes and form adhesions. Voleti and colleagues[4] state that preventing and limiting adhesions can be accomplished by limiting trauma, decreasing inflammatory response via pharmacologic agents, or the introduction of mechanical barriers between the tendons and proliferating tissue.

The use of tendon grafts and wraps to facilitate glide and prevent adhesions is a controversial topic. Although commercial corporations have made several types of wraps and attest to their usefulness, many surgeons think that the wraps increase bulk and do not prevent adhesions. Exploring individual grafts is outside the scope of this article; however, nonsponsored literature on the subject is not readily available.

FIXATION TECHNIQUES

With the advances in technology over the past decade, fixation options have changed dramatically. Although the previous techniques are still functional, the advances in medical supplies have helped increase pull-out strength, decrease needed dissection and exposure, and decrease operative time. In general, the transfer can be secured via tenodesis with another tendon or secured to osseous structures directly. When a tendon is fixated to another tendon, different suture techniques are available to increase the overall strength and vascularity to the transferred tendon. A side-to-side tenodesis is the simplest technique but can result in suture slippage and loss of fixation. The Pulvertaft weave is a technique where the transferred tendon is woven through tunnels in the recipient tendon multiple times and sutured together. The 2 tendons can be combined in a spiral technique, where the donor tendon is twisted together with the recipient and sutured together. A double-loop technique and a lasso double-loop technique can be used where a loop is formed from each tendon and they are combined. The loop techniques are stronger but have increased overall bulk.[7,8,16,22] Suture anchors are also available on the market and consist of many different nonabsorbable and absorbable anchors with sutures connected to them to secure the tendon to the desired structure.

Tendon to osseous fixation can be performed using several different techniques, all of which result in final fixation via ossification of the tendon to the bone after healing. This can be accomplished by making a bone tunnel, which the tendon passed through. The tendon can be secured by suturing the tendon back on to itself and using interference screws or trephine bone plugs. Sutures used to pass the tendon through the osseous tunnel can be passed through the other side of the foot and a button placed on the outside of the skin. With the button technique, there is concern for tissue necrosis in the area of the button, so placing a barrier with gauze or foam between the button and the cutaneous tissue is beneficial. Alternative fixation techniques consist of a screw and washer technique; the tendon can be sutured directly to the periosteum as well.[8,16]

POSTOPERATIVE CONSIDERATIONS

When a patient leaves the operating room, the treatment is just beginning. Casting and postoperative dressings can be beneficial or harmful. Immobilization is necessary to prevent elongation of the transfer, traumatic rupture of the transfer, or failure of the fixation in the initial postoperative period.[13,23] Many patients requiring a transfer in the lower extremity have concomitant sensory defects that could result in overaggressive ROM in the initial postoperative period; therefore, these patients and the repair must be protected. The healing process of a tendon transfer creates a delicate rehabilitation process because the tendon insertion must have time to heal, but the longer an area remains static the more likely it is to contract and adhere.

Immobilization

Postoperatively, adhesions occur, but they should be beneficial to the repair and not detrimental. The first priority in the postoperative period is healing of the incision and tendinous structures, prior to concern about adhesions. The time frame for immobilization varies depending on the surgery performed, the surgeon, and the patient. Neuropathic patients and patients with poor tissue quality may require longer periods of immobilization than another healthier patient.

Rehabilitation Process

Once a tendon has had adequate time to heal at its new insertion point, rehabilitation and physical therapy can begin. This is a long process for some patients, and communication between surgeon and therapist is vital. Rehabilitation begins with gentle passive ROM exercises that mimic the movements the tendon are responsible for creating. After weeks of passive ROM and partial immobilizations (controlled ankle movement boots, braces, and so forth), protected active ROM can begin. This is when gait and proprioception are concentrated on. Lastly is strength training; this is often the period when patients are freed of any devices and begin to increase muscle mass. This should be a slow and steady process under the guidance of a therapist for several weeks or months.

SUMMARY

Medicine and surgery are ever-evolving fields. As new techniques emerge, the old techniques are often forgotten. It is important to build on current concepts and knowledge of anatomy. Other investigators will closely scrutinize specific surgeries, but keep in mind the close parallels in technique despite the different desirable outcomes. Tendon transfers can provide large amounts of correction whether used alone or in conjunction with other procedures. Understanding how to properly execute a tendon transfer can be an invaluable skill for any surgeon.

REFERENCES

1. Fenton C, Gilman D, Jassen M, et al. Criteria for selected major tendon transfers in podiatric surgery. J Am Podiatry Assoc 1983;73(11):561–8.
2. Hoard A, Bell-Krotoski J, Mathews R. Application of biomechanics to tendon transfers. J Hand Ther 1995;8:115–23.
3. Connizzo B, Bhatt P, Liechty K, et al. Diabetes alters mechanical properties and collagen fiber re-alignment in multiple mouse tendons. Ann Biomed Eng 2014; 42(9):1880–8.
4. Voleti P, Buckley M, Soslowsky L. Tendon healing repair and regeneration. Annu Rev Biomed Eng 2012;14:47–71.
5. O'Brien M. Functional anatomy and physiology of tendons. Clin Sports Med 1992; 11(3):505–20.
6. Frey C, Shereff H, Greenidge N. Vascularity of posterior tibial tendon. J Bone Joint Surg Am 1990;72:884–6.
7. McGlamry ED, Joe TS. Principles of muscle-tendon surgery and tendon transfers. McGlamry's comprehensive textbook of foot and ankle surgery. 4th edition. Philadelphia: Wolters Kluwer Health/Lippincott Williams & Wilkins; 2013. p. 1127–64.
8. Peljovich A, Ratner J, Marino J. Update of the physiology and biomechanics of tendon transfer surgery. J Hand Surg 2010;35:1365–9.
9. Friden J, Ponten D, Lieber R. Effect of muscle tension during tendon transfer on sarcomerogenesis in a rabbit model. J Hand Surg 2000;25A:138–43.
10. Friden K, Lieber R. Evidence for muscle attachment at relatively long lengths in tendon transfer surgery. J Hand Surg 1998;23A:105–10.
11. Koh T, Herzog W. Excursion is important in regulating sarcomere number in the growing rabbit tibialis anterior. J Physiol 1998;508:267–80.
12. Hoffer M. The use of the pathokinesiology laboratory to select muscles for tendon transfers in the cerebral palsy hand. Clin Orthop Relat Res 1993;288:135–8.
13. Sammers D, Chung K. Tendon transfers: Part 1. Principles of transfer and transfers for radial nerve palsy. Plast Reconstr Surg 2009;123(5):169–77.
14. Fessel G, Snedeker J. Evidence against proteoglycan mediated collagen fibril load transmission and dynamic viscoelasticity in tendon. Matrix Biol 2009;28(8): 503–10.

15. Perry J, Hoffer M. Preoperative and postoperative dynamic electromyography as an aid in planning tendon transfers in children with cerebral palsy. J Bone Joint Surg Am 1977;59(4):531–7.
16. Fitoussi F, Bachy M. Tendon lengthening and transfer. Orthop Traumatol Surg Res 2015;101:s149–57.
17. Silver RL, de la Garza J, Rang M. The myth of muscle balance. A study of relative strengths and excursion of normal muscles about the foot and ankle. J Bone Joint Surg Br 1985;67(3):432–7.
18. Lieber R, Brown C. Quantitative method for comparison of skeletal muscle architectural properties. J Biomech 1992;25(5):557–60.
19. Boahene K. Principles and biomechanics of muscle tendon unit transfer: application in temporalis muscle tendon transposition for smile improvement in facial paralysis. Laryngoscope 2012;123:350–5.
20. Giurintano D. Basic biomechanics. J Hand Ther 1995;8:79–84.
21. Dykyj D, Jules K. The clinical anatomy of tendons. J Am Podiatr Med Assoc 1991; 81(7):358–65.
22. Vigasio A, Marcoccio I, Patelli A, et al. New tendon transfer for correction of drop-foot in common peroneal nerve palsy. Clin Orthop Relat Res 2008;466:1454–66.
23. Grauwin M, Wavreille G, Fontaine C. Double tendon transfer for correction of drop-foot. Orthop Traumatol Surg Res 2015;101(1):115–8.

Flexor Digitorum Longus Tendon Transfer and Modified Kidner Technique in Posterior Tibial Tendon Dysfunction

CrossMark

James T. Maskill, DPM[a],*, Gregory C. Pomeroy, MD[b]

KEYWORDS

- Posterior tibial tendon dysfunction (PTTD) • Kidner procedure
- Flexor digitorum longus tendon • Flatfoot

KEY POINTS

- Isolated tendon transfers or soft-tissue procedures by themselves are generally reserved for stage 1 posterior tibial tendon dysfunction (PTTD).
- When a modified Kidner procedure or flexor digitorum longus tendon transfer is used in stage 2 PTTD, it should be supplemented with osseous procedures.
- Tendon transfers are contraindicated for stage 3 PTTD.

INTRODUCTION

Posterior tibial tendon dysfunction (PTTD) is a well-known cause of painful flatfoot affecting persons of all ages. In 1989 Johnson and Strom were the first to describe PTTD in 3 different stages.[1] Stage 1 is described as posterior tibial tendonitis, with no significant deformity in the hindfoot. Treatment is largely targeted toward conservative management, although tenosynovectomy or flexor digitorum longus transfer may be considered if conservative treatment fails.[2,3] Stage 2 is consistent with a flexible flatfoot deformity whereby the posterior tibial tendon (PTT) is elongated. The treatment of stage 2 flatfoot remains controversial for both conservative and surgical management. Stage 3 is an arthritic and, therefore, rigid flatfoot that can be treated with bracing and orthotics to prevent further progression of the valgus deformity.[4] However, if conservative management fails, surgical correction would be indicated, which would include hindfoot arthrodesis.[5] Stage 4 was described by Myerson,[6]

[a] Orthopaedic Associates of Kalamazoo, 3810 Center Avenue, Portage, MI 49024, USA;
[b] University of New England, 195 Fore River Parkway Suite 210, Portland, ME 04102, USA
* Corresponding author.
E-mail address: Jtmaskil1@gmail.com

Clin Podiatr Med Surg 33 (2016) 15–20
http://dx.doi.org/10.1016/j.cpm.2015.06.007
0891-8422/16/$ – see front matter © 2016 Elsevier Inc. All rights reserved.

and is characterized by the same findings in stage 3 with the addition of ankle valgus deformity and arthritis of the ankle joint. The flexor digitorum longus tendon transfer and modified Kidner procedure are commonly used when treating the early stages of PTTD, and are often used in conjunction with a combination of osteotomies to correct the flatfoot deformity if present.

MODIFIED KIDNER PROCEDURE

In 1933, Kidner[7] was the first to describe the procedure whereby the accessory navicular was removed from the PTT and the PTT was reattached to the undersurface of the navicular body with sutures. He noted that interruption of the insertion of the PTT through the accessory navicular is associated with increased prevalence of dysfunction of the PTT. Since then there have been modifications, including bone anchors, drill holes into the navicular, and biotenodesis screws, which have been proved to produce reliable pain relief and patient satisfaction.[8–10] It also has been described in the pediatric population to simply excise the accessory navicular, leaving the PTT intact.[11] Diagnosis can be made by physical examination, whereby often the accessory navicular is more prominent and, at times, painful. Weight-bearing foot radiographs are used to confirm the diagnosis and are needed preoperatively. If there is uncertainty of the presence of an accessory navicular or the condition of the PTT, advanced imaging such as MRI and computed tomography may be indicated.[12] This procedure is best used for stage 1 and 2 PTTD.

Operative Technique

The patient is placed supine on the operating table. A padded thigh tourniquet is then placed, and the affected lower extremity is prepared and draped in the usual sterile fashion. The limb is then exsanguinated, and the tourniquet is inflated. Attention is then directed to the medial hindfoot, where a 5-cm incision is made starting from the tip of the medial malleolus to just past the insertion of the PTT. The PTT sheath is then opened and traced distally to the navicular tuberosity (**Fig. 1**A). The PTT is then sharply dissected off the navicular. The tendon should always be inspected for any tendinopathy, and be addressed accordingly (see **Fig. 1**B). Next the accessory navicular is shelled out from the posterior tibial tendon, leaving healthy tendon behind (see **Fig. 1**C). An oscillating saw can then be used to resect any excess navicular tuberosity to create a cancellous bed for reattachment of the PTT (see **Fig. 1**D). A bone anchor is then placed into the navicular body at the level of the PTT insertion. Care needs to be taken not to place the bone anchor into the talonavicular joint or the naviculocuneiform joint (NCJ) (see **Fig. 1**E). Alternatively, drill holes may be placed into the navicular, creating a tunnel for the tendon. The tendon is then tightly secured to the cancellous bone. It is important to hold the ankle at neutral dorsiflexion and foot in neutral abduction/adduction during the placement of the posterior tibial tendon into the main body of the navicular (see **Fig. 1**F). The tendon should be placed under slight tension, accomplished by advancing it on the navicular. If the plantar accessory insertions of the PTT have been violated, they should be reapproximated to the advanced tendon (see **Fig. 1**G). The wound is then closed, and a Jones compressive dressing and posterior sugar tong splint are applied with the ankle at 90°.

Postoperative Course

The senior author prefers the patient to remain non–weight bearing for 8 weeks. Skin staples are removed at the 2-week point. Patient will transition to a short leg

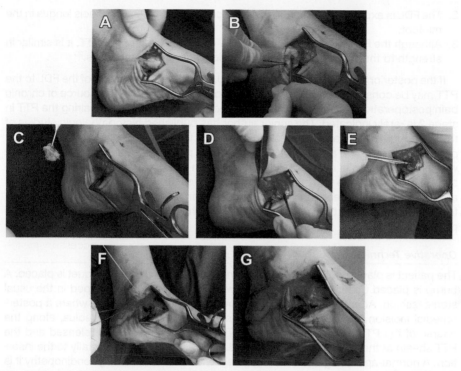

Fig. 1. Modified Kinder procedure. (*A*) Posterior tendon and the navicular tuberosity. (*B*) Accessory navicular in the PTT. (*C*) Accessory navicular completely excised. (*D*) Cancellous bed at the navicular tuberosity. (*E*) Bone anchor placed into the navicular body at the level of the PTT insertion. (*F*) PTT tendon advanced onto the navicular with the ankle at neutral dorsiflexion and foot in neutral abduction/adduction. (*G*) PTT securely advanced onto the navicular.

non–weight-bearing fiberglass cast for an additional 6 weeks. After 8 weeks the patient will transition to normal shoe gear and gradually return to full activities.

FLEXOR DIGITORUM LONGUS TENDON TRANSFER

Flexor digitorum longus (FDL) transfer has been described for stage 1 and 2 PTTD. In stage 1 disease the PTT needs to be explored if conservative management fails. If there is abnormality in the substance of the tendon, it should be debrided accordingly to healthy tendon.[6,13,14] In this instance an FDL transfer can be considered to support the function of the PTT.[14–16] The authors do not advocate this in every case, as sacrificing the FDL would leave the surgeon with limited options for tendon transfer in stage 2 disease.

In stage 2 disease, the PTT has become permanently elongated and attenuated with longitudinal tears, although the flatfoot remains flexible.[13,17–20] FDL tendon transfer alone is never indicated in stage 2 PTTD, as it must be supported with corrective bony osteotomies to supplement the tendon transfer.[3,13,15] The FDL tendon transfer is an excellent option for stage 2 flatfoot, for multiple reasons:

1. The FDL is adjacent to the PTT and courses behind the medial malleolus; therefore, they have the same line of pull, and this is an in-phase tendon transfer.

2. The FDL is expendable because of its attachment to the flexor hallucis longus in the midfoot.
3. Although the FDL has approximately 30% of the strength of the PTT, it is similar in strength to the antagonist of the PTT, which is the peroneal brevis.[21]

If the posterior tibial tendon can be repaired, a side-to-side transfer of the FDL to the PTT may be considered. Leaving the diseased PTT intact could be a source of chronic pain postoperatively, despite correction of the flatfoot deformity. Repairing the PTT in stage 2 is rarely indicated. The senior author has published histopathologic studies of the PTT in stage 2 disease, which clearly show the tendon is not viable.[18,20,21] Often on physical examination, the examiner can feel the posterior tibial tendon and palpate whether the tendon is normal, thickened, or even ruptured. Advanced Imaging such as MRI can be used to further evaluate the PTT if desired.[12] Routine foot radiographs are usually all that is needed for preoperative planning for correction of a stage 2 flatfoot. The FDL tendon transfer for stage 2 PTTD has been proved to be reliable and predicable.[14–16,22,23]

Operative Technique

The patient is placed supine on the operating table, and a thigh tourniquet is placed. A bump is placed under the affected limb, which is prepared and draped in the usual sterile fashion. Attention is then directed toward the medial hindfoot, where a posteromedial incision is made starting just posterior to the medial malleolus, along the course of the PTT, to the NCJ (**Fig. 2**A). The flexor retinaculum is released and the PTT sheath at the medial malleolus incised. The tendon is traced distally to the insertion. A normal-appearing PTT has a light yellow color. If there is any tendinopathy it is usually located on the undersurface, is usually a pale white color and often bulbous, and the fibrillar nature disappears. Often the tendon has ruptured (see **Fig. 2**B).[16,18] If there are no signs of disease, a side-to-side transfer may be considered. If the PTT is diseased, it is resected (see **Fig. 2**C). The FDL tendon sheath is then identified and located just deep to the PTT (see **Fig. 2**D). The FDL is traced distally through the knot of Henry, then tenotomized and brought into the wound. Care should be taken to avoid violating the medial plantar neurovascular bundle. There is often enough harvested to transfer the FDL tendon to the medial cuneiform. Transferring the tendon to the medial cuneiform rather than the navicular may serve as support at the NCJ, where it often sags.[24] Just distal to the NCJ 2 drill holes are then made, 1 inferior and 1 superior, creating a tunnel in the body of the cuneiform (see **Fig. 2**E–G). A Kessler-type stitch is then placed into the distal stump of the FDL tendon with 0 Ethibond suture. The tendon is then passed through the tunnel (see **Fig. 2**H, I). The length of the stump is enough to bring the tendon into the tunnel and often long enough to bring it into the superior aspect of the tunnel. With the foot held inverted and plantarflexed, the FDL tendon stump is sewn into the anterior tibialis tendon that lies adjacent to the superior hole. This maneuver will allow for a secure anchor. The FDL is then reinforced with adjacent soft tissues on the plantar surface of the cuneiform and navicular (see **Fig. 2**J). If the harvested tendon does not have sufficient length or there is no collapse at the NCJ, a bone anchor may be placed into the navicular to secure the FDL tendon appropriately to the bone. The wound is then closed, and a Jones compressive dressing and posterior sugar tong splint are applied.

Postoperative Course

The senior author prefers the patient to remain non–weight bearing for 8 weeks. Skin staples are removed after 2 weeks. The patient will transition to a short leg

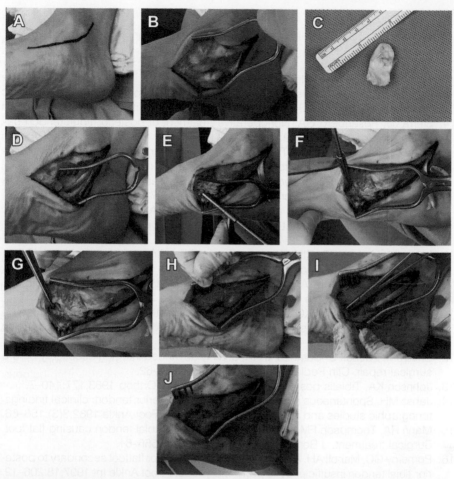

Fig. 2. (*A*) Posteromedial incision starting just posterior to the medial malleolus to the na-viculocuneiform joint. (*B*) Diseased, thickening, and ruptured posterior tibial tendon. (*C*) Excised posterior tibial tendon. (*D*) FDL tendon. (*E*) Plantar medial aspect of the medial cune-iform. (*F*) Superior aspect of the medial cuneiform. (*G*) Tunnel created in the medial cunei-form to pass the FDL tendon. (*H*) Kessler-type stick placed into the stump of the FDL tendon. (*I*) Passing the FDL tendon inferior to superior through the created tunnel in the medial cuneiform. (*J*) FDL tendon fully secured and reinforced with adjacent soft tissues on the plantar surface of the cuneiform and navicular.

non–weight-bearing fiberglass cast for an additional 6 weeks. After 8 weeks the pa-tient will transition to normal shoe gear and gradually return to full activities.

SUMMARY

PTTD is a painful disease that is often progressive. The use of tendon transfers should be reserved for stage 1 or 2 disease when the deformity is still supple. When deformity is present, soft-tissue procedures alone are not sufficient to completely correct the flatfoot. Therefore, osseous procedures are often used to supplement the soft-tissue procedures. These tendon transfers have proved to be reliable and predictive when used for PTTD, also in combination with appropriate bony osteotomies.

REFERENCES

1. Johnson KA, Strom DE. Tibialis posterior tendon dysfunction. Clin Orthop Relat Res 1989;(239):196–206.
2. Teasdall R, Johnson KA. Surgical treatment of stage 1 posterior tibial tendon dysfunction. Foot Ankle Int 1994;12:646–8.
3. Funk DA, Cass JR, Johnson KA. Acquired adult flat foot secondary to posterior tibial tendon pathology. J Bone Joint Surg Am 1986;68:95–101.
4. Sferra JJ, Rosenberg GA. Nonoperative treatment of posterior tibial tendon pathology. Foot Ankle Clin 1997;2:261–73.
5. Graves SC, Stephenson K. The use of subtalar and triple arthrodesis in the treatment of posterior tibial tendon dysfunction. Foot Ankle Clin 1997;2:319–28.
6. Myerson MS. Adult acquired flatfoot deformity. Treatment of dysfunction of the posterior tibial tendon. J Bone Joint Surg Am 1996;78:780–92.
7. Kidner FC. The prehallux in relation to flatfoot. JAMA 1933;101:1539–42.
8. Lee KT, Kim KC, Park YU, et al. Midterm outcome of modified Kidner procedure. Foot Ankle Int 2012;33:122–7.
9. Kopp FJ, Marcus RE. Clinical outcome of surgical treatment of the symptomatic accessory navicular. Foot Ankle Int 2004;25:27–30.
10. Micheli LJ, Nielson JH, Ascani C, et al. Treatment of painful accessory navicular: a modification to simple excision. Foot Ankle Spec 2008;1:214–7.
11. Cha SM, Shin HD, Kim KC, et al. Simple excision vs the Kidner procedure for type 2 accessory navicular associated with flatfoot in pediatric population. Foot Ankle Int 2013;34:167–72.
12. Baca JM, Zdenek C, Catanzariti AR, et al. Is advanced imaging necessary before surgical repair. Clin Podiatr Med Surg 2014;31:357–62.
13. Johnson KA. Tibialis posterior tendon rupture. Clin Orthop 1983;177:140–7.
14. Jahss MH. Spontaneous ruptures of the tibialis posterior tendon: clinical findings, tenographic studies and a new technique of repair. Foot Ankle 1982;3(3):158–66.
15. Mann RA, Thompson FM. Rupture of the posterior tibial tendon causing flat foot. Surgical treatment. J Bone Joint Surg Am 1985;67:556–61.
16. Pomeroy GC, Manoli AH. A new operative approach for flatfoot secondary to posterior tibial tendon insufficiency: a preliminary report. Foot Ankle Int 1997;18:206–12.
17. Gazdag AR, Cracchiolo A. Rupture of the posterior tibial tendon. Evaluation of injury of the spring ligament and clinical assessment of tendon transfer and ligament repair. J Bone Joint Surg Am 1997;79:675–81.
18. Mosier SM, Lucas DR, Pomeroy GC, et al. Pathology of the posterior tibial tendon in posterior tibial tendon insufficiency. Foot Ankle Int 1998;19:520–4.
19. Mann RA. Rupture of the tibialis posterior tendon. Instr Course Lect 1984;33: 302–9.
20. Mann RA, Coughlin MJ. Surgery of the foot and ankle. 6th edition. St Louis (MO): Mosby; 1993.
21. Silver RL, Garza J, Rang M. The myth of muscle balance. J Bone Joint Surg Br 1985;3(67):432–7.
22. Shereff M. Treatment of ruptured posterior tibial tendon with direct repair and FDL tenodesis. Foot Ankle Clin 1997;2:281–96.
23. Myerson MS, Corrigan J, Thompson F, et al. Tendon transfer combined with calcaneal osteotomy for treatment for posterior tibial tendon insufficiency: a radiological investigation. Foot Ankle Int 1995;16:712–8.
24. Hansen ST. Functional reconstruction of the foot and ankle. Philadelphia: Lippincott Williams & Wilkins; 2000.

Tibialis Anterior Tendon Transfer for Posterior Tibial Tendon Insufficiency

Crystal L. Ramanujam, DPM, MScª, John J. Stapleton, DPMb,c,
Thomas Zgonis, DPMd,*

KEYWORDS

- Tibialis anterior tendon • Flatfoot • Posterior tibial tendon dysfunction • Cobb
- Calcaneal osteotomy • Surgery

KEY POINTS

- The Cobb procedure is useful for addressing stage 2 posterior tibial tendon dysfunction.
- The Cobb procedure is usually accompanied by a medial displacement calcaneal osteotomy and/or lateral column lengthening.
- The Cobb procedure can also be combined with selected medial column arthrodesis and realignment osteotomies along with equinus correction when indicated.

INTRODUCTION

The role of posterior tibial tendon (PTT) dysfunction (PTTD) as a cause of adult-acquired flatfoot is well established. Johnson and Strom's[1] classification of PTTD separated the flexible from the rigid deformities and provided recommended surgical treatments for each stage. In the early stages of PTTD (stage 1 and stage 2), when the condition is flexible, soft tissue reconstructive procedures can be used to achieve pain relief and prevent progression to rigid deformity. Stage 2 PTTD encompasses a wide range of clinical manifestations; therefore, several surgical procedures have been proposed for correction of an insufficient or elongated PTT in combination with a supple hindfoot valgus after failed nonoperative management. To date, the most commonly reported procedures used to correct stage 2 PTTD are the flexor digitorum longus

ª Division of Podiatric Medicine and Surgery, Department of Orthopaedics, University of Texas Health Science Center at San Antonio, 7703 Floyd Curl Drive MSC 7776, San Antonio, TX 78229, USA; b Foot and Ankle Surgery, VSAS Orthopaedics, Lehigh Valley Hospital, 1250 S Cedar Crest Boulevard, Suite # 110, Allentown, PA 18103, USA; c Penn State College of Medicine, 500 University Drive, Hershey, PA 17033, USA; d Division of Podiatric Medicine and Surgery, Department of Orthopaedic Surgery, University of Texas Health Science Center San Antonio, 7703 Floyd Curl Drive MSC 7776, San Antonio, TX 78229, USA
* Corresponding author.
E-mail address: zgonis@uthscsa.edu

Clin Podiatr Med Surg 33 (2016) 21–28
http://dx.doi.org/10.1016/j.cpm.2015.06.002
0891-8422/16/$ – see front matter © 2016 Elsevier Inc. All rights reserved.

tendon (FDLT) transfer in combination with medial displacement calcaneal osteotomy (MDCO) and/or lengthening of the lateral column. Although these techniques may correct the loss of the medial arch and forefoot abduction, supination deformity of the forefoot is not addressed; this can become more problematic for patients with correction of the hindfoot.[2] In addition, alternative transfer using the tibialis anterior tendon (TAT) has been proposed to avoid sacrificing the FDLT because it plays such a key role in the biomechanical function of the foot.[3]

HISTORICAL PERSPECTIVE

In 1923, Lowman[4] reported the use of the TAT as a sling under the navicular to restore the medial arch in symptomatic flatfeet. In the late 1970s, Cobb[5] described a technique for stage 2 PTTD using a split tibialis anterior musculotendinous graft to reconstruct the PTT, restore plantar flexion function of the first ray, and correct forefoot supination. The original Cobb procedure included first a medial incision to expose the damaged PTT for resection and then a second incision over the anterior muscle compartment proximal to the ankle for splitting of the TAT. The anterior half of the anterior tendon is then passed distally in its sheath and through a drill hole in the medial cuneiform into the PTT sheath across the site of the PTT deficit and then secured at the plantar surface of the naviculocuneiform (NC) joint with the healthy proximal portion of the PTT. Since its inception, the Cobb procedure, with certain modifications, has been described by Helal, Benton-Weil and Weil, and Janis and colleagues.[6–8] Each of these investigators provided overviews of their modifications in a small number of patients. Since then, several larger series have been published on the outcomes of the TAT transfer in combination with other corrective procedures for the treatment of symptomatic stage 2 PTTD, which provide more detailed information and longer follow-up (**Table 1**).

INDICATIONS

The Cobb procedure is mostly used for stage 2 PTTD. The acquired flatfoot deformity must be flexible and corrected at the time of the Cobb procedure. Often, an MDCO is performed to address the calcaneal valgus and to realign the weight-bearing axis of the heel with the tibia. In addition, if significant midfoot/forefoot abduction is present, it may be addressed with lateral column lengthening. At times, compensatory forefoot varus may be present; if not addressed, it can lead to destabilization of the medial column and recurrent rear foot deformity. Forefoot varus is best approached with a first tarsometatarsal (TMT) arthrodesis as opposed to a Cotton opening wedge osteotomy with bone grafting when a Cobb procedure is performed. The inherent stability of the TMT arthrodesis corrects the forefoot varus while providing additional stability to the medial longitudinal arch. In addition, a drill hole can still be placed through the medial cuneiform for passage of the split portion of the TAT if desired. Gastrocnemius recession or percutaneous tendo-Achilles lengthening in the presence of equinus may also need to be corrected before any realignment procedures. Significant advantages of the Cobb procedure are that tendon function is not sacrificed and it provides a suspensory effect to the medial column of the foot. In select cases, the Cobb procedure can be used to reconstruct the spring ligament in conjunction with an FDLT transfer (**Fig. 1**).

COBB TECHNIQUE

An approximately 3-cm incision is placed over the proximal anterolateral portion of the TAT. The retinaculum is released; the medial half portion of the TAT is identified, split,

Table 1
Case series involving Cobb procedure for stage 2 PTTD

Authors, Year	N	Age Range	Adjunct Procedures	Average Follow-up	Postoperative Outcome	Complications
Giorgini et al,[9] 2010	50 Feet in 39 patients	5–70 y	Kidner procedure (resection of accessory navicular and/or prominent navicular tuberosity with advancement of PTT insertion)	4.6 y	48 Good (no pain, unlimited activity, no difficulty with shoe fit) 2 Fair (occasional pain, limit on strenuous activity, minor difficulty with shoe fit)	1 Wound dehiscence 1 Fractured hardware
Parsons et al,[10] 2010	32 Feet in 32 patients	44–66 y	Medial displacement translational osteotomy of calcaneus	5.1 y	Mean AOFAS hindfoot score of 89 29 Were able to perform single-heel rise test (none before surgery) at 12 mo and final follow-up All preferred to wear comfort insoles in normal footwear	1 Superficial wound dehiscence 1 Temporary dysesthesia of medial plantar nerve
Madhav et al,[11] 2009	43 Feet in 43 patients	27–75 y	Rose calcaneal osteotomy (transverse osteotomy with excision of medially based one-half width wedge of bone)	4.28 y	Mean AOFAS hindfoot score of 85 66% Were able to perform single-heel rise test 78% Were able to use normal footwear 65% No longer required orthotics	1 Saphenous nerve injury 1 Sural nerve injury 4 Cases of oozing from wounds 2 Developed subtalar joint osteoarthritis 6 Cases required screw removal for local irritation

(continued on next page)

Table 1
(continued)

Authors, Year	N	Age Range	Adjunct Procedures	Average Follow-up	Postoperative Outcome	Complications
Knupp & Hintermann,[2] 2007	22 Feet in 22 patients	29–64 y	Deltoid ligament reconstruction (17 patients) Spring ligament repair (3 patients) Medial sliding calcaneal osteotomy (11 patients) Calcaneal lengthening osteotomy (3 patients)	2.0 y	Mean AOFAS hindfoot score of 88.5 86% Were able to wear shoes without modifications or orthotics 14% Preferred to have orthotic inlays	1 Skin necrosis 1 Loss of sensation at the medial aspect of the midfoot 2 Patients had revision surgery because of pain (1 triple arthrodesis and 1 screw removal)
Weil et al,[12] 1998	13 Feet in 13 patients	53–80 y for stage 2 PTTD and 41–73 y for stage 3 PTTD	Cobb reconstruction alone in stage 2 PTTD (5 patients) Evans lateral column lengthening (8 patients)	1.0 y–5.25 y	Patients with stage 2 PTTD had a better satisfaction than patients with stage 3	1 Patient in stage 2 PTTD did not meet expectations. and half of the patients in stage 3 PTTD did not meet expectations

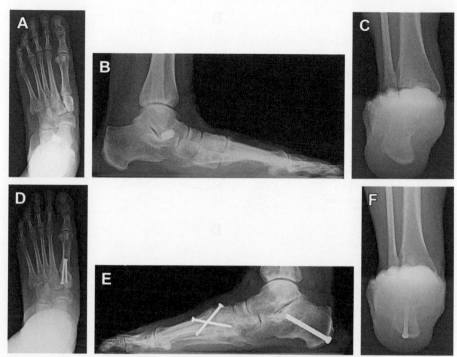

Fig. 1. Preoperative anteroposterior (*A*), lateral (*B*), and calcaneal axial (*C*) views of a previous multiple surgical reconstructions of the PTT with synovectomy, tendon allografting, and subtalar joint arthroereisis. Patient underwent revision reconstructive surgery with removal of the subtalar joint implant, MDCO, lateral column lengthening, first TMT joint arthrodesis, FDLT transfer, and Cobb procedure. Final postoperative radiographs (*D–F*) at 1-year follow-up.

and kept in place by an umbilical tape while maintaining its insertion on the medial cuneiform. A large curved hemostat or tendon passer is then introduced from distal to proximal orientation and under the TAT sheath to exit at the proximal leg incision. The umbilical tape is then introduced to the tendon passer and exits distally at the insertion of the TAT to the medial cuneiform. At that time the TAT can be split, and after it is released proximally. The harvested portion of the TAT can then be passed under the periosteum or through a drill hole in the medial cuneiform. A transfer and tenodesis of the split portion of the TAT is then performed with the remaining portion of the PTT after it was debrided. The tenodesis should be performed with the foot held in a plantar-flexed and inverted position. The Cobb procedure can also be combined with an FDLT transfer when the posterior tibialis muscle excursion is compromised and the spring ligament is attenuated. It is also preferable to perform the Cobb procedure after all osteotomies and selected arthrodesis sites have been completed (**Fig. 2**).

ADJUNCTIVE PROCEDURES
Medial Displacement Calcaneal Osteotomy

MDCO is performed to correct the hindfoot valgus deformity, assist in medialization of the Achilles tendon, and to reestablish the weight-bearing hindfoot alignment axis of the calcaneus with the tibia. The MDCO aligns the foot into a more mechanically advantageous position, thus offsetting the load on the tendon transfer. The osteotomy is

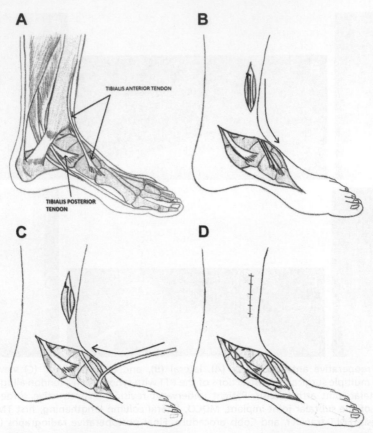

Fig. 2. Tendon and osseous anatomy with location of the TAT and PTT (*A*). Incision placements for access to pathologic PTT for debridement and for harvesting of split medial half of the TAT with arrow depicting direction of tendon separation (*B*). Arrow depicts direction of rerouting the split TAT graft along its tendon sheath to its most distal attachment at the medial cuneiform and base of the first metatarsal (*C*). The TAT graft placed through a drill hole into the medial cuneiform and then with the foot placed in plantar flexion and inversion; the tendon graft is then weaved through and attached to the distal end of the PTT (*D*).

performed through a direct 4- to 5-cm oblique incision located posterior and inferior to the peroneal tendons and course of the sural nerve. Blunt dissection is taken down to the lateral calcaneal wall, and an oblique osteotomy is performed with an oscillating saw with caution to avoid overpenetrating the medial calcaneal wall. The osteotomy is distracted with lamina spreaders stretching the medial periosteum to allow for displacement. The osteotomy is then translated medially approximately 1 cm or based on the alignment desired. Distal translation can be performed to increase the calcaneal pitch. The osteotomy can be secured with a single 6.5-mm cannulated screw or other various methods of fixation.

Lateral Column Lengthening

The main goal of the lateral column lengthening is to correct abduction of the midfoot and forefoot. This procedure can provide triplane correction of an acquired flatfoot deformity by the mechanical advantage of the peroneal longus to correct forefoot varus resulting in compensatory varus position of the calcaneus. The lateral column lengthening is often combined with an MDCO. The double osteotomy allows correction of acquired hindfoot valgus and forefoot/midfoot abduction deformity. A 3-cm longitudinal incision is made directly over the floor of the sinus tarsi and anterior process of the calcaneus. The sural nerve and the peroneal tendons are identified and retracted accordingly. A sagittal saw is used to create an osteotomy approximately 1.5 cm proximal to the calcaneocuboid joint. The osteotomy is distracted, and a piece of tricortical bone graft is used to achieve the lengthening. This osteotomy may or may not be secured with any type of fixation.

First Tarsometatarsal Arthrodesis

When medial column stabilization and/or correction of forefoot varus are required in conjunction with a Cobb procedure, it is advantageous to include an arthrodesis of the first TMT joint. Indications for a first TMT include significant forefoot varus, abnormal lateral talo-first metatarsal angle on weight-bearing lateral radiographs, TMT joint arthrosis, first metatarsal elevatus, and/or hypermobility of the medial column. In addition the incision over the first TMT joint allows exposure of the distal TAT. The first TMT joint is exposed through a 5-cm incision fashioned just medial to the extensor hallucis longus tendon over the TMT joint. Meticulous joint preparation

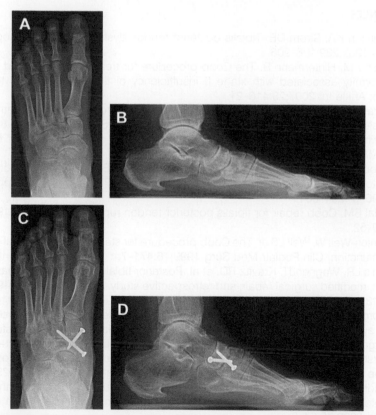

Fig. 3. Preoperative anteroposterior (*A*) and lateral (*B*) views of a stage 2 PTTD that underwent a combined Cobb procedure with a naviculocuneiform arthrodesis. Final postoperative radiographs (*C, D*) at approximately 1-year follow-up.

is required to avoid nonunion. The first metatarsal is plantar flexed, and fixation is generally performed with dual-compression lag screws.

Naviculocuneiform Arthrodesis

In certain cases, whereby medial column stabilization is required in conjunction with the Cobb procedure, an NC arthrodesis may be performed in the presence of NC joint arthrosis, instability, and sagging. The surgical incision also provides exposure of the distal portion of the TAT for the Cobb procedure, and arthrodesis is achieved with compression lag screws (**Fig. 3**).

SUMMARY

The Cobb procedure may be considered for stage 2 PTTD in conjunction with realignment osteotomies and/or selected medial column stabilization arthrodesis procedures. Although retrospective in nature, the collective findings of the studies in **Table 1** demonstrate that the Cobb procedure is a useful technique to decrease pain and improve function for stage 2 PTTD. Although it is difficult to analyze the effects of the adjunct procedures performed in the aforementioned studies, a randomized control trial that directly compares the Cobb procedure plus MDCO with the FDLT transfer plus MDCO would be beneficial.

REFERENCES

1. Johnson KA, Strom DE. Tibialis posterior tendon dysfunction. Clin Orthop Relat Res 1989;239:196–206.
2. Knupp M, Hintermann B. The Cobb procedure for treatment of acquired flatfoot deformity associated with stage II insufficiency of the posterior tibial tendon. Foot Ankle Int 2007;28:416–21.
3. Baravarian B, Zgonis T, Lowery C. Use of the Cobb procedure in the treatment of posterior tibial tendon dysfunction. Clin Podiatr Med Surg 2002;19:371–89.
4. Lowman CL. An operative method for the correction of certain forms of flatfoot. JAMA 1923;81:1500–2.
5. Cobb N. Tibialis posterior tendon disorders. In: Helal B, Rowley DI, Cracchiola A, editors. Surgery of disorders of the foot and ankle. Philadelphia: JB Lippincott; 1996. p. 291–301.
6. Helal BM. Cobb repair for tibialis posterior tendon rupture. J Foot Surg 1990;29: 349–52.
7. Benton-Weil W, Weil LS Jr. The Cobb procedure for stage II posterior tibial tendon dysfunction. Clin Podiatr Med Surg 1999;16:471–7.
8. Janis LR, Wagner JT, Kravitz RD, et al. Posterior tibial tendon rupture: classification, modified surgical repair, and retrospective study. J Foot Ankle Surg 1993;32: 2–13.
9. Giorgini R, Giorgini T, Calderaro M, et al. The modified Kidner-Cobb procedure for symptomatic flexible pes planovalgus and posterior tibial tendon dysfunction stage II: review of 50 feet in 39 patients. J Foot Ankle Surg 2010;49:411–6.
10. Parsons S, Naim S, Richards PJ, et al. Correction and prevention of deformity in type II tibialis posterior dysfunction. Clin Orthop Relat Res 2010;468:1025–32.
11. Madhav RT, Kampa RJ, Singh D, et al. Cobb procedure and Rose calcaneal osteotomy for the treatment of tibialis posterior tendon dysfunction. Acta Orthop Belg 2009;75:64–9.
12. Weil LS Jr, Benton-Weil W, Borrelli AH, et al. Outcomes for surgical correction for stages 2 and 3 tibialis posterior dysfunction. J Foot Ankle Surg 1998;37:467–71.

Posterior Tibial Tendon Transfer

Amber M. Shane, DPM, FACFAS[a,b,*], Christopher L. Reeves, DPM, MS, FACFAS[b,c], Jordan D. Cameron, DPM[d], Ryan Vazales, DPM[e]

KEYWORDS

- Equinovarus • Posterior tibial tendon transfer • PTTT • Tendon transfer
- Posterior tibial tendon • Dropfoot

KEY POINTS

- Proper tensioning of the tendon is key to maintaining the greatest amount of strength available from the transferred tendon.
- Patient education of rehabilitation and out-of-phase tendon training is paramount for success.
- Interosseous technique is recommended as opposed to the circumtibial route, creating a generous window in the membrane to allow for free movement of the tendon.
- Assurance of proper muscle strength and grade must be evaluated preoperatively to achieve success.
- Adequate tendon length must be demonstrated before passing the transfers.

INTRODUCTION

Tendon balancing using the posterior tibial tendon for the correction of a deforming drop foot disorder is both common and complex. It is a procedure that is often indicated in high-risk patients presenting with multiple comorbidities. Complications range in severity and depend on the underlying pathophysiology (flaccid paralytic

Financial Disclosure: The authors have nothing to disclose as it relates to the content of this article.
Conflict of Interest: Nothing to report.
[a] Orlando Foot and Ankle Clinic, 250 North Alafaya Trail, Suite 115, Orlando, FL 32825, USA; [b] Department of Podiatric Surgery, Florida Hospital East Orlando Surgical Residency Program, 7727 Lake Underhill Road, Orlando, FL 32822, USA; [c] Orlando Foot and Ankle Clinic, 2111 Glenwood Drive, Suite 104, Winter Park, FL 32792, USA; [d] Podiatric Medicine and Surgery Resident (PGY-2), Florida Hospital East Orlando Residency Training Program, 7727 Lake Underhill Road, Orlando, FL 32822, USA; [e] Podiatric Medicine and Surgery Resident (PGY-1), Florida Hospital East Orlando Residency Training Program, 7727 Lake Underhill Road, Orlando, FL 32822, USA
* Corresponding author. Orlando Foot and Ankle Clinic, 250 North Alafaya Trail, Suite 115, Orlando, FL.
E-mail address: ambershanereeves@yahoo.com

disorders vs spastic cerebral palsy) of the deforming force and degree of flexibility. Rigid osseous deforming forces have been seen to coexist with soft tissue involvement, and when not corrected, often limit the tendon balancing effectiveness. This is because anatomic joint excursion under passive range of motion is decreased with tendon transfers. Perioperative management should include correcting osseous deformities before or in conjunction with tendon procedures and is paramount to a successful result. Patient education and the capacity of the patient to undergo extensive functional rehabilitation and muscle retraining are essential to achieve activate dorsiflexion during the swing phase of gait.[1] The ultimate goal of the tibialis posterior tendon transfer is to create a stable plantigrade foot thereby correcting the deforming force leading to inefficiency and/or instability during walking.[2] The hope is to obviate the need for an ankle foot orthosis or plantarflexion-limiting brace; however, patients should be aware that permanent bracing could be required, depending on whether the tendon transfer is functional versus a static sling, as well as the ability for other major muscle groups and intrinsic muscles to stabilize stance.

In 1937, Mayer discussed 5 principles of tendon transfer.[3] These 5 principles are paramount in obtaining a successful tendon transfer procedure. These principles include restoration of the anatomic relationship between a tendon and its sheath, tendon routing through the tissue that allows for gliding, restoring normal tendon tension, re-creation of the anatomic tendon insertion, and establishing a proper line of tendon pull.[3] In-phase tendon transfers are often thought of as the preferred, most effective, and efficient method. Out-of-phase transfers require greater length of retraining and therapy. It has been proposed that out-of-phase tendon transfers act solely as a static restraint to the deformity.[4,5]

The functions of the tendon, as well as the distance of the tendon from the joint axis, are important points to consider when planning a tendon transfer. The function of the tendon can be determined by its position in relation to the site or joint that is being considered. The distance from the joint is what determines the lever arm of force that can be applied across the joint. These musculotendinous structures work in pairs to counterbalance one another. They become antagonists to each other, allowing for the pull of one tendon to oppose that of the corresponding tendon. When one of these components becomes weak or loses its ability to function, a deformity is created owing to the antagonistic muscle/tendon. This becomes a key point when determining which tendon is to be transferred and to where it should be transferred.

Normal tension on the tendon is an important consideration when performing a tendon transfer. Studies show that fixating a tendon with too much or too little tension can lead to the tendon becoming ineffective.[6,7] Blix curve shows us that it is desired to have the tendon midway between maximal length and the relaxed position to allow it to generate the most effective pull.[8] This length allows for optimal myofilament overlap, which creates the maximal amount of force. Friden, in a study on upper extremity tendon transfers, found that using passive tension as a guide for the optimal length often results in overstretching of the sarcomeres, resulting in a loss of muscle strength.[7] Overtensioning, as opposed to undertensioning, is often the preferred technique for many surgeons when fixating a tendon that is transferred owing to the thought that the repair site may slip or stress–relax. However, relying on the repair site to relax or slip is not a recommended method owing to the fact it will often result in loss of strength.

ANATOMY AND BIOMECHANICS

Under normal physiologic conditions, the primary function of the tibialis posterior muscle/tendon (PTT) through its multiple attachments on the plantar aspect of the foot are supination of the subtalar joint, adduction of the midfoot, and plantarflexion of the ankle.[2] The firing of the PTT occurs solely in stance phase of normal gait. Eccentric firing of the muscle begins after heel strike allowing pronation of the hindfoot to occur. This causes an unlocking mechanism to the talonavicular and calcaneal cuboid joints, providing the foot with the ability to absorb shock. Continued concentric firing of the PTT in midstance and toe off phases of gait effectively function to supinate the hindfoot and lock and lock the talonavicular and calcaneal cuboid joints to create a rigid lever for the gastroc/soleus complex to drive push off of the forefoot.[9] As such, a PTT transfer is unique among other transfers because, upon transfer of the tendon, the muscle/tendon not only changes its' direction of action to dorsiflexion, but does so during an entirely separate phase of gait, the swing phase.

Not only is a tendon's ability to perform a needed action important in transfer, but its strength before transfer is also a key factor in successful outcomes. Studies have shown that, when transferring a tendon, the surgeon must take into account an expected associated loss of a grade of strength. Therefore, it is imperative that the tendon in question be strong and healthy before transfer. A study by Silver and colleagues[10] looked at relative muscle strength of tendons as proportional to cross-sectional area and found the PTT to be stronger than any of the other primary tendons in the foot including the tibialis anterior, peroneus longus, peroneus brevis, flexor hallucis, and flexor digitorum. This increased strength of the PTT allows for minimizing morbidity of the functionality of tendon during transfer allowing it to be a versatile choice of treatment and correction of multiple paralytic disorders.

INDICATIONS

Originally, posterior tibial tendon transfer was used to treat flaccid paralytic disorders such a poliomyelitis and leprosy, as presented by Watkins in 1954.[11] However, since that time, the indications for the procedure has broadened to include supinated equinovarus deformities secondary to clubfoot, mononeuropathy, peroneal nerve palsies,[12] progressive drop foot disorders like Charcot Marie Tooth disease, and even spastic disorders like cerebral palsy.[13] These conditions alter balance, quality of gait, and decrease the ability to accomplish activities of daily living.[14] Operative intervention can alleviate these problems, as well as reduce the necessity of an orthosis in many cases. In cases of nerve trauma, a window of 18 to 24 months should be allowed before any operative intervention to allow a window for possible recovery with conservative treatment.[15]

PREOPERATIVE CONSIDERATIONS

Before electing to perform PTT transfer, several factors need to be evaluated to ensure an optimal outcome. First, the etiology of the deformity must be determined. Is the deformity static or progressive? In some instances, the deformity has a rigid component and the tendon transfer must be performed in conjunction with an arthrodesis or realignment osteotomy procedures. A Coleman block test can be used to determine if the heel is flexible or rigid and aids in the surgical decision-making process.

Another factor to consider is the strength of the everters of the foot, the peroneal muscle group. A large concern when performing a PTT transfer is the possibility of developing an inversion deformity. In 2013, Das and colleagues[16] studied peroneal strength as a determining factor for selecting a route for the tendon transfer. They found that peroneal strength did, in fact, play a role in preventing inversion deformity. When determining to use a circumtibial route it was found that the patient should have peroneal muscle strength of 4 or higher. This begs the question that if the muscle strength is

4 or higher is there a true necessity to perform a tendon transfer or if the problem can be managed with other treatment modalities. Those that have peroneal muscle strength of 3 or lower it is recommended to use the interosseous membrane approach.[16]

We typically obtain nerve conduction studies and EMGs during surgical planning. These will allow the surgeon to choose the optimal procedure based on the patient's specific pathology. In cases where muscle strength is minimal, the procedure can still function as a tenodesis (or static "stirrup") to reduce the drop foot deformity despite a lack of dorsiflexion being present.[17]

Patients must be educated on the expectation of range of motion preoperatively and postoperatively and about the need for in-depth physical therapy to return to a more normal gait pattern. Physical therapy includes training the PTT to dorsiflex during the swing phase of gait. This action is most often accomplished with voluntary control and rarely does this occur as an involuntary physiologic response. A patient should expect to use his or her brace or ankle foot orthosis for approximately 6 months after the procedure.[17] It is important that the patient have a proper knowledge of the postoperative plan to prevent him or her from becoming discouraged.

PROCEDURE THEORY

Since its infancy, the transfer of the posterior tibial tendon has had an incorporation of many modifications; however, there has yet to be any research that proves any 1 procedure superior to the next.[18–20] The procedure was originally described by Watkins and colleagues in 1954, in which the PTT transfer is rerouted through the interosseous membrane and anchored to the dorsal lateral aspect of the foot. Common modifications noted in the literature include techniques involving 3 incisions verses 4 and the passing of the tendon either over or under the retinaculum. Theoretically, the greater the distance a tendon is from a joint axis, the greater the force that it exerts across the joint as a result of a longer lever arm. This, combined with preoperative assessment and postoperative expectations of the patient, play an important role when determining whether to pass a tendon beneath the retinaculum or subcutaneously. When one pursues a transfer beneath the retinaculum, common in the 4-incision technique, the tendon is closer to the joint. This diminishes the lever arm and muscle strength, but increases tendon range of motion, potentially providing more dorsiflexion capability. The opposite holds true for subcutaneous placement; the tendon is further from the joint meaning an increased lever arm. This phenomenon is represented by the Blix curve, which describes the relationship of muscle length and contractile force.[15] It has also been found that the interosseous technique has a lesser incidence of recurrent inversion deformities. There has been a satisfactory finding when evaluating the improvement in gait and prevention of trophic changes with this technique as well, whereas the circumtibial route has been associated with a high rate of recurrent inversion, which can lead to ulceration of the lateral foot border.[21]

Regardless of the number of incisions or placement of the tendon above or below the retinaculum, the surgeon should place the tendon that he or she is transferring at zero tension (physiologic tension), midway between completely relaxed and maximum length. Zero tension is achieved when the foot is in the desired position without any slack. Surgeons frequently place tendons in slightly greater tension because there is a degree of muscle stretching that can take place.

OPERATIVE TECHNIQUE

The patient is positioned supine about the operating table. Should a tourniquet be needed, a thigh application would be most suitable; however, many surgeons opt to perform the procedure without one because correct anatomic dissection and well-placed incisions are adequate to control regional bleeding.[1] The affected lower extremity including the thigh and lower leg foot and ankle are scrubbed, prepped, and draped in standard aseptic technique. General anesthesia is often accompanied with a popliteal block. The author prefers a 4-incision approach (medial foot, medial leg, anterior leg, and dorsal foot; **Fig. 1**). The first medial incision is placed parallel to the course of the PTT between the medial malleolus and dorsal aspect of the navicular bone approximately 3 to 4 cm in length. Dissection is carried down to the tendon sheath and the tendon is isolated circumferentially. When harvesting the tendon, maintenance of tendon length is paramount. Place the belly of the scalpel blade parallel and lateral to the tendon and tease the tendon away from the navicular bone as distal as possible. The tendon can then be isolated and harvested as far distal as possible as it courses plantar to the midfoot. The distal end can then debrided and tabularized to prepare for implantation. It is recommended to apply a temporary whip-stitch as this point to maintain distal control of the tendon when attempting the proximal medial harvest (**Fig. 2**). The next incision is completed to the medial lower leg in line with the posterior–medial border of the tibia bone and 1 cm posterior to it. The center of this incision is approximately 15 cm proximal to the distal tip of the medial malleolus. The incision is deepened to the fascia and upon opening the fascia the first structure identified is the flexor digitorum longus muscle belly. Fascial components are teased away and the muscle is retracted anteriorly. Deep to the flexor digitorum longus is the posterior tibial tendon. Place tension on the distal aspect of the posterior tibial tendon while visualizing the tendon to ensure that it is in fact the correct tendon. Tease the muscle belly away from its facial components and protect the posterior neurovascular bundle. The tendinous portion of the muscle belly will be visualized and is the easiest structure to add proximal tension to and carefully deliver the entire PTT through the 3- to 4-cm proximal incision (**Figs. 3** and **4**). Many surgeons currently use tendon passers to complete this task. Once the entire tendon has been gathered proximally, a third incision is then made on the anterior surface of the lower leg at the level of the intersection of the middle and distal third and approximately 1 cm lateral to the tibial crest. This incision should be distal to the proximal medial incision to facilitate passage of tendon and improve the functionality of the transfer. To allow good exposure and easy passage of the PTT, the incision is often larger than the other 3 measuring approximately 4 to 6 cm in length. The tibialis anterior muscle belly is visualized through this incision and is separated and retracted medial. This maneuver provides visualization to the interosseous membrane (**Figs. 5** and **6**). Blunt dissection is completed and the neurovascular bundle and the remaining musculature are retracted laterally. The interosseous membrane is visualized. Posterior to the interosseous

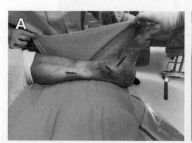
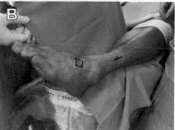

Fig. 1. (*A* and *B*) Surgical incision planning showing proposed locations for incisions.

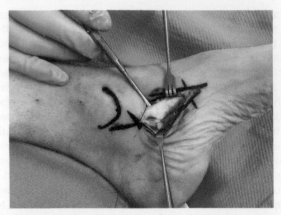

Fig. 2. Harvesting of the posterior tibial tendon from the insertion site.

membrane is the posterior neurovascular bundle. As a result, it is safest to open the membrane from the posterior side so as to not plunge instrumentation posteriorly. The authors prefer to use a right angle forceps and carefully "ride" the posterior tibia through the medial leg incision. This technique allows for protection of the bundle. The tips forceps are then rotated anteriorly and carefully used to puncture the interosseous membrane. Blunt opening of the membrane is performed until there is approximately a 4-cm, longitudinal opening of the membrane. Again, staying in contact with the posterior tibia, the tendon is passed form the medial incision, through the interosseous membrane, and delivered anteriorly. Optimally, the PTT muscle belly should extend through the interosseous window to prevent adhesions (**Fig. 7**). Finally, after marking out the anatomy of the foot via fluoroscopy, a fourth incision is completed over the lateral cuneiform measuring approximately 2 to 3 cm in length. A tendon passer or instrument of similar function (eg, Bozeman forceps, Ober tendon passer, tendon transfer wire, or aortic clamp) is retrograded through the incision and deep to the retinaculum and accepts the PTT and draws it distally (**Fig. 8**). The authors prefer to anchor the tendon into the lateral cuneiform with a through and through osseous tunnel technique and tenodesis screw for fixation. However, there have been multiple

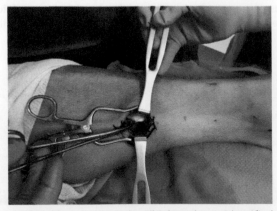

Fig. 3. From the second incision the posterior tibial tendon is identified.

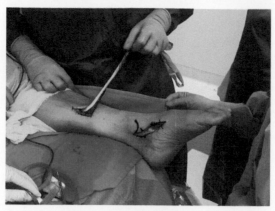

Fig. 4. The posterior tibial tendon is then pulled through the distal leg and out of the second incision.

modifications to this technique in the form of location of the transfer as well as fixation (**Figs. 9** and **10**).[22,23]

A second technique for this procedure has also been described whereby there are only 3 incisions used; the medial lower leg incision is not used.[24] One further technique modification was described by Srinivasan and colleagues[25] in 1968, whereby the tendon was split longitudinally into "2 tails" a medial and a lateral, which were then tenodesed to the extensor halluces longus and extensor digitorum longus and peroneus tertius accordingly thereby avoiding the possible varus or valgus deformity postoperatively.

Regardless of the number of incisions, during the anchoring phase of the tendon, the knee should be flexed and the ankle should be dorsiflexed to neutral position. This is to take into account the smaller excursion of the PTT compared with the tendons it is replacing. The lesser excursion often leads to decreased ankle range of motion and therefore increased dorsiflexion at time of anchor is suggested.

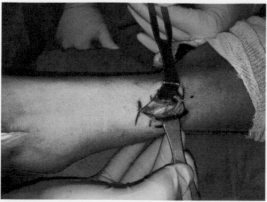

Fig. 5. The third incision, lateral to the tibia with visualization of the interosseous membrane.

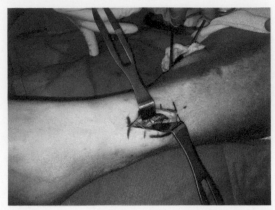

Fig. 6. A hemostat is passed from the second incision to the third incision and visualized in the interosseous membrane.

POSTOPERATIVE CARE

Patients are placed in a cast or posterior splint following the procedure with care taken to keep the foot held in a dorsiflexed position. The patient is kept in a cast for 2 to 4 weeks, allowing enough time for the incision sites to be fully healed. After 3 weeks, or once the incision sites are healed, gentle passive range of motion exercises are initiated.[21] During the range of motion exercises, plantar flexion is avoided initially until approximately 6 weeks. This is done to avoid any excess force being placed on the newly transferred tendon. From 6 to 10 weeks, partial weight bearing may be initiated with the use of a walking boot.[17] It has been found that Sharpey's fibers, type III collagen, were present and connected at the tendon–bone interface by 6 weeks.[26] Extensive physical therapy is needed as the posterior tibial tendon is an out-of-phase tendon transfer, which requires the patient to relearn the swing phase of walking. This process can be very extensive and require long-term physical therapy for this to become involuntary. During the early phases of rehabilitation, conscious effort is needed to dorsiflex the foot. Less concentration is needed months after the

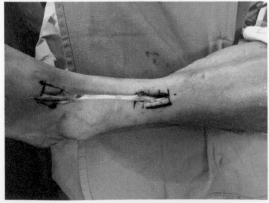

Fig. 7. The tendon is then passed through the window in the membrane and removed through the third incision.

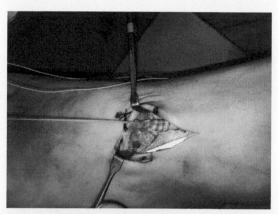

Fig. 8. Through the fourth incision on the dorsum of the foot, the tendon is pulled below the retinaculum. The site of the anchor has been drilled according to the size of the tendon.

tendon transfer. Between 6 and 12 months postoperatively, no conscious effort is needed to actively dorsiflex using the PTT.[26] Communication and education of patients is key, because patients will not be brace free for a period of at least 6 months after surgery.[17]

COMPLICATIONS

Despite all the advances and changes in techniques, these variations in procedure techniques still carry similar risks. One commonly reported problem is that of loss of inversion of the foot.[17] Many of the newer methods have been developed to help prevent this specific problem. Clawing of the toes is also a possible complication or undesired outcome. Clawing often happens as a result of suturing to the extensor digitorum tendon.[21] As a result, this technique is not commonly used or recommended. A common concern is the development of a flatfoot deformity owing to the removal and loss of the posterior tibial tendon. This does frequently occur; however, it occurs with a more normal gait pattern indicating that the body weight was being

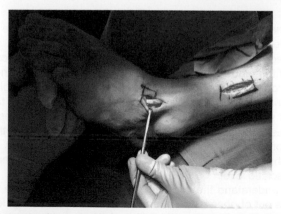

Fig. 9. The tendon inserted into the dorsum of the foot with the foot placed in the desired position to allow for proper tensioning.

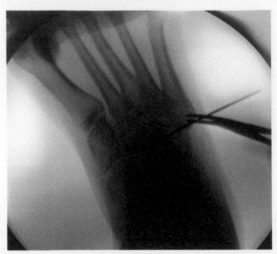

Fig. 10. Intraoperative fluoroscopy showing the desired location, in this instance to insert the tendon in the midfoot.

more equally and evenly distributed. A transfer of the flexor digitorum longus tendon to the PTT insertion site has been used to help prevent collapsing of the arch in select cases. Bowstringing of the tendon can occur if the tendon is not passed below the retinaculum. There are multiple techniques that involve passing the tendon above the retinaculum; in these cases, the bowstringing effect should be discussed with the patient. Recurrence of the initial problem is always a risk when performing any soft tissue procedure; however, there has not been overwhelming evidence of this in the literature. Another issue that may be encountered intraoperatively is a tendon that is too short to reach its designated implantation site. When this occurs, one can first attempt to rectify the problem by increasing the size of the intraosseous membrane tunnel. Should this not rectify the issue looking for alternative implantation sites is analyzed. Other cuneiforms, cuboid, and more commonly the talar neck can be used if necessary. A last resort is tendon lengthening or tenodesis to the long extensor tendons.

DISCUSSION

Key principles when performing tendon transfers include retaining the normal relationship between the transplanted tendon and the gliding apparatus. Minimal trauma should be inflicted, avoid injury to the sheath, paratenon, and delicate gliding cells on the surface of the tendon that can be caused by improper handling of the tendon. Last, establish proper mechanical lines of traction to allow the transplanted tendon to have the appropriate mechanical advantage to perform the desired task.

Proper patient selection and preparation will allow for optimal results. One study found that men less than 30 years old had much better results than others who underwent the same procedure. The same study found greater success when the nerve lesion causing the drop foot was at the level of the common peroneal nerve as opposed to the sciatic level.[27]

Patients must understand the need for physical therapy after the procedure. This tendon transfer is out of phase, which requires extensive retraining, leading to the ultimate goal of a plantigrade gait pattern. Transferring any tendon causes a 1-grade loss in muscle strength, so any dysfunction before the procedure will be amplified.

Occasionally, there can be a loss in plantarflexory power as well. This was noted to affect those with proximal nerve lesions, with minimal effect to those with common peroneal nerve lesions.[27]

When performed correctly with the right patient population, a PTT transfer is an effective procedure. Many different methods have been established for fixating the tendon, each of which has its' own indications. Passing through the interosseous membrane is the preferred and recommended method and should be used unless this is not possible.[21] Good surgical planning based on patient needs and expectations, along with excellent postoperative care including early range of motion and physical therapy minimizes risk of complications and allows for the optimal outcome to be achieved.

REFERENCES

1. Landsman A, Cook E, Cook J. Tenotomy and tendon transfer about the forefoot, midfoot and hindfoot. Clin Podiatr Med Surg 2008;25:547–69.
2. Aronow MS. Tendon transfer options in managing the adult flexible flatfoot. Foot Ankle Clin N Am 2012;17:205–26.
3. Mayer LM. The physiological method of tendon transplantation in the treatment of paralytic drop-foot. J Bone Joint Surg 1937;19:389–94.
4. Mann RA. Tendon transfers and electromyography. Clin Orthop Relat Res 1972; 85:64–6.
5. Waters R, Frazier J, Garland D. Electromyograghic gait analysis before and after operative treatment for hemiplegic equinus and equinovarus deformity. J Bone Joint Surg Am 1982;64:284–8.
6. Blix M. Die lange und die spannug des muskels. Skand Arch Physiol 1894;5: 149–206.
7. Friden J, Lieber RLP. Evidence for muscle attachments at relatively long lengths in tendon transfer surgery. J Hand Surg 1998;23(1):105–10.
8. Schweitzer KM, Jones CPM. Tendon transfers for the drop foot. Foot Ankle Clin N Am 2014;19:65–71.
9. Bluman E, Dowd T. The basics and science of tendon transfers. Foot Ankle Clin 2011;16:385–99.
10. Silver R, De La Garza J, Rang M. The myth of muscle balance: a study of relative muscle strengths and excursions of normal muscles about the foot and ankle. J Bone Joint Surg Br 1985;67:432–7.
11. Watkins M, Jones JB, Ryder CT Jr, et al. Transplantation of the posterior tibial tendon. J Bone Joint Surg Am 1954;36:1181–9.
12. Pinzur M, Kett N, Trilla M. Combined anteroposterior tibial tendon transfer in post traumatic peroneal palsy. Foot Ankle 1988;8:271–5.
13. Root L, Miller S, Kirz P. Posterior tibial-tendon transfer in patients with cerebral palsy. J Bone Joint Surg Am 1987;69:1133–9.
14. Gasq DM, Molinier FM, Reina NDPP, et al. Posterior tibial tendon transfer in the spastic brain-damaged adult does not lead to valgus flatfoot. J Foot Ankle Surg 2013;19:182–7.
15. DiDomenico LD, Cane LD. Key insights on tendon transfers for drop foot. Podiatry Today 2009;(5):22.
16. Das P, Kumar J, Karthikeyan GSRP. Peroneal strength as an indicator in selecting route of tibialis posterior transfer for foot drop correction in leprosy. Lepr Rev 2013;84:186–93.
17. Richardson DR, Gause NLM. The bridle procedure. Foot Ankle Clin N Am 2011; 16:419–33.

18. Rodriguez R. The bridle procedure in the treatment of paralysis of the foot. Foot Ankle 1992;13:63–9.
19. Prahinski J, McHale K, Temple HT, et al. Bridle transfer for paresis of the anterior and lateral compartment musculature. Foot Ankle Int 1996;17:615–9.
20. Wagenaar F, Lowerens J. Posterior tibial tendon transfer: results of fixation the dorsiflexors proximal the ankle joint. Foot Ankle Int 2007;28:1128–42.
21. Shah RK. Tibialis posterior transfer by interosseous route for the correction of foot drop in leprosy. Int Orthop 2009;33:1637–40.
22. Mulier T, Rummens E, Dereymaeker G. Risk of neurovascular injuries in flexor hallucis longus tendon transfers: an anatomic cadaver study. Foot Ankle Int 2007;28: 910–5.
23. Southerland J, Boberg J, Downey M, et al. McGlamry's comprehensive textbook of foot and ankle surgery. Philadelphia: Wolters Kluwer Health/Lippincott Williams & Wilkins; 2013.
24. Turner J, Cooper R. Anterior transfer of the tibialis posterior through the interosseous membrane. Clin Orthop 1972;79:71–4.
25. Srinivasan H, Mukherjee S, Subramaniam R. Two-tailed transfer of tibialis posterior for correction of drop-foot in leprosy. J Bone Joint Surg Br 1968;50:623–8.
26. Jeng CM, Myerson MM. The uses of tendon transfers to correct paralytic deformity of the foot and ankle. Foot Ankle Clin N Am 2004;9:319–37.
27. Yeap JS, Birch R, Singh D. Long-term results of tibialis posterior tendon transfer for drop-foot. Int Orthop 2001;25:114–8.

Tibialis Anterior Tendon Transfer

Jennifer L. Mulhern, DPM[a], Nicole M. Protzman, MS[b],
Stephen A. Brigido, DPM[a],*

KEYWORDS

- Clubfoot • Equinovarus deformity • Split tibialis anterior tendon transfer • STATT
- Tendon transfer • Tibialis anterior tendon

KEY POINTS

- For successful tendon transfer, appropriate patient selection and detailed preoperative examination are paramount.
- The surgeon must consider any underlying pathologies, fully evaluate the strength of the tibialis anterior muscle, and perform the appropriate concomitant procedures.
- Tibialis anterior tendon transfers are most successful in reducible deformities. If a nonreducible deformity is present, transfer must be combined with other procedures.
- Complete and split tibialis anterior tendon transfers are a well-accepted method of treatment for idiopathic equinovarus deformities.
- Research has confirmed the effectiveness of both the complete and split transfer of the tibialis anterior tendon to restore muscle balance and improve functional autonomy.

INTRODUCTION

Tendon transfer procedures have long been used for the correction of complex foot deformities in adults and children. Because many deformities coexist, however, concomitant bony and soft tissue procedures are often necessary for successful correction. Transfer of the tibialis anterior tendon is used commonly to treat recurrent clubfoot and to restore muscle balance in patients with cerebral palsy. Recurrent clubfoot deformities are often attributable to an overactive tibialis anterior muscle and weak antagonists. Although many techniques have been proposed for the correction

Disclosure Statement: Dr S.A. Brigido serves on the surgery advisory board for Alliqua and Bacterin International. He also serves as a consultant for Stryker, Zimmer and Wright Medical. None of the aforementioned companies had any knowledge or influence on study design, protocol or data collection. For the remaining authors, no potential conflicts of interest exist.
[a] Foot and Ankle Department, Foot and Ankle Reconstruction, Coordinated Health, 2775 Schoenersville Road, Bethlehem, PA 18017, USA; [b] Clinical Education and Research Department, Coordinated Health, 3435 Winchester Road, Allentown, PA 18104, USA
* Corresponding author.
E-mail address: drsbrigido@mac.com

Clin Podiatr Med Surg 33 (2016) 41–53
http://dx.doi.org/10.1016/j.cpm.2015.06.003
0891-8422/16/$ – see front matter © 2016 Elsevier Inc. All rights reserved.

of recurrent clubfoot deformities, the most common treatments include the complete and split transfer of the tibialis anterior tendon.

Complete transposition of the anterior tibial tendon was first described by Garceau in 1940[1,2] and later modified by Ponseti. The Ponseti technique popularized and is largely accepted as the standard treatment for the management of idiopathic clubfoot.[3,4] The technique aims to correct dynamic supination by transferring the tibialis anterior tendon laterally.

Several decades later, the split tibialis anterior tendon transfer (STATT) was introduced by Hoffer and colleagues.[5] The STATT is a variation of the complete tibialis anterior tendon transfer where the tibialis anterior tendon is split and the lateral half is secured into the lateral cuneiform or cuboid. When initially introduced, the STATT procedure was used to treat children with cerebral palsy and spastic equinovarus deformity. Since then, the indications have expanded to include the treatment of residual clubfoot deformity as well as spastic equinovarus deformity in adults.[5–7] As with the complete transfer of the tibialis anterior tendon, the STATT procedure attempts to neutralize the varus pull of the tibialis anterior muscle.[8] Both the complete and split transfers have proven safe and effective means of achieving deformity correction, restoring muscle balance, and improving functional autonomy.[6,9] The present report discusses the key aspects of both the complete transfer of the tibialis anterior tendon and the STATT, including the operative indications and contraindications, key aspects of preoperative planning, operative techniques and rehabilitation protocols, and lastly, published outcomes are reviewed.

Pathomechanics

Weak evertors allow the tibialis anterior muscle to have an unopposed pull creating a dynamic supination of the forefoot.[10] Transferring the tendon laterally balances inversion and eversion and reduces the talo-first metatarsal angle.[11]

Indications

Successful outcomes depend on appropriate patient selection. **Table 1** outlines the indications for both the tibialis anterior tendon transfer and the STATT.

Contraindications

There are very few absolute contraindications to tibialis anterior tendon transfer. The procedure should be avoided when muscle strength of the tibialis anterior is less than 4+ or 5[15] and when severe contraction limits tendon length and prevents the transfer

| Table 1 | |
Indications for tibialis anterior tendon transfer and split tibialis anterior tendon transfer	
Tibialis Anterior Tendon Transfer	**Split Tibialis Anterior Tendon Transfer**
Spastic rearfoot varus[12,13]	Recurrent clubfoot[10,12–14]
Spastic equinovarus[12,13]	Flexible forefoot equinus[12,13]
Excessive inversion power[12]	Dynamic forefoot supinatus[13]
Forefoot equinus with swing-phase extensor substitution[12]	Dropfoot[12]
Flexible cavovarus[12]	Tarsometatarsal amputation[12]
Excessive supination in gait[12]	Charcot–Marie–Tooth deformity[12,14]
Dorsiflexor weakness[12]	

In rigid deformity indications, the tendon transfer should be performed in conjunction with bony procedures.
Data from Refs.[10,12–14]

of the distal end laterally.[16] In rigid deformities, the procedure should not be performed in isolation.

SURGICAL TECHNIQUE
Preoperative Planning

Detailed preoperative planning is critical to proper deformity correction. The information garnered can be used to identify the underlying pathology as well as the origin and cause of the deformity. As part of the preoperative planning process, a thorough patient history and clinical examination should be conducted. The patient's pain, sensory deficits, and ambulatory status should be taken into consideration. The clinical examination should include both a static evaluation of foot position and a dynamic evaluation with gait analysis. Tools are available to enhance the study of patient biomechanics. For example, dynamic pedobarography can be employed to measure the pressure distribution patterns during gait, instrumented 3-dimensional gait analysis provides visualization of foot movements in all 3 planes, and electrophysiologic examination can assist in the detection of muscle or nerve dysfunction.

Muscle strength of the tibialis anterior must be accurately quantified. An initial strength of 4+ or greater is required to retain functionality, as one grade of muscle strength is typically lost following tendon transfer (**Table 2**).[15] Weight-bearing lateral and anteroposterior radiographs of the foot and ankle should be obtained. In cases of severe deformity, additional studies, such as magnetic resonance imaging or computed tomography, may be necessary to evaluate the deformity fully. These imaging modalities will allow the surgeon to identify any superimposed bony deformities that may require correction during the index procedure.[14]

Kuo and colleagues[17] suggest that the most appropriate point of fixation is the lateral cuneiform in the full tendon transfer and the cuboid bone in the split tendon

Table 2
Evaluation of muscle strength. A 4+/5 or a 5/5 muscle strength is required for successful transfer

Grade	Muscle Activity
5	Normal power; maximal resistance
4+	Full range of motion: can overcome gravity and almost full resistance
4	Full range of motion: can overcome gravity and moderate resistance
4−	Full range of motion: can overcome gravity and mild resistance
3+	Full range of motion: can overcome gravity and slight resistance
3	Full range of motion: can overcome gravity only
3−	Full range of motion: can overcome partial gravity only
2+	Partial range of motion against gravity or complete range of motion, gravity eliminated, while holding against minimal resistance
2	Full range of motion: gravity eliminated
2−	Partial range of motion: gravity eliminated
1	No visible motion; palpable contraction
0	No motor activity

Data from Kendall FP, McCreary EK, Provance PG, et al. Fundamental concepts. In: Lappies P, editor. Muscles: testing and function, with posture and pain. 5th edition. Baltimore (MD): Lippincott Williams & Wilkins; 2005. p. 1–48; and Hislop HJ, Avers D, Brown M. Principles of manual muscle testing. In: Duncan L, editor. Daniels and Worthingham's Muscle testing: techniques of manual examination and performance testing. 9th edition. St Louis (MO): Elsevier Saunders; 2013. p. 1–11.

transfer. This is not a hard-and-fast guideline, because selection of the anchoring bone is based on clinical evaluation, particularly the strength of the peroneals and the amount of correction necessary to balance the foot. The greater the correction, the more laterally the fixation must be placed.

As stated by Lampasi and colleagues,[11] "in feet with a rigid or partially correctable deformity, transfer of the [tibialis anterior tendon] should not be expected to provide much improvement, except for reduction of adduction in more flexible feet, and correction should be provided by other procedures." For this reason, the transfer of the tibialis anterior tendon is rarely performed in isolation. Most commonly, a gastrocnemius recession is required to address equinus deformity.[12,13] If spasticity of the posterior tibial tendon exists, a myotendinous lengthening may be necessary to reduce associated heel varus.[18] Fixed deformities may require calcaneal osteotomy, subtalar or triple arthrodesis, extensor tendon lengthening, or tenotomies for digital correction. These procedures should always be considered during the preoperative evaluation.

Despite an overwhelming acceptance of the procedure, there is no defined temporal indication. It is generally agreed that transfer of the tendon alone or with a gastrocnemius recession may be more effective in children, whereas bony procedures are often required in older patients. In any event, a comprehensive operative approach is needed, tailored specifically to the deformity and the patient.

Preparation and Patient Positioning

Patient positioning must permit exposure to the medial foot, lateral foot, and anterior leg. Therefore, the patient should be supine with an ipsilateral bump to position the leg rectus with the tibial tuberosity forward. A combination of general and regional anesthesia is preferred, but spinal anesthesia can also be used. A pneumatic thigh tourniquet is insufflated after exsanguination of the lower leg.

Operative Approach

A 3-incision approach is used for both the tibialis anterior tendon transfer and the STATT, with incision placement as follows (**Fig. 1**):

1. Dorsal–medially on the foot overlying the tibialis anterior tendon insertion at the medial side of the medial cuneiform and base of the first metatarsal;

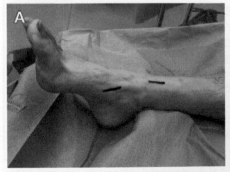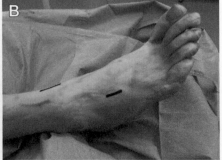

Fig. 1. Incision placement for transfer of the tibialis anterior tendon. Incisions 1 and 2 provide exposure to the tendon (A), whereas incision 3, located laterally on the dorsal aspect of the foot, represents the point of tendon stabilization (B). The technique shown provides stabilization through fixation into the lateral cuneiform.

2. Anteriorly within the lower leg, just proximal to the extensor retinaculum; and
3. Dorsal–laterally on the foot, overlying the lateral cuneiform or cuboid.

Operative Procedure

Tibialis anterior tendon transfer

The sheath is incised in a linear fashion (incision 1; (**Fig. 2**)). The tendon is identified and sharply released from its insertion. Through the incision on the anterior leg (incision 2), the tibialis anterior tendon is identified and gently pulled proximally along its sheath through the incision. The end of the tendon is "tagged" with a suture in a whip-stitch fashion. A tendon passer is inserted through the dorsal-lateral foot incision (incision 3), and retrieved through the anterior leg (incision 2). Care must be taken to ensure that the tendon passer remains within the long extensor sheath, underneath the extensor retinaculum. The tendon is retrieved and delivered through the dorsal–lateral

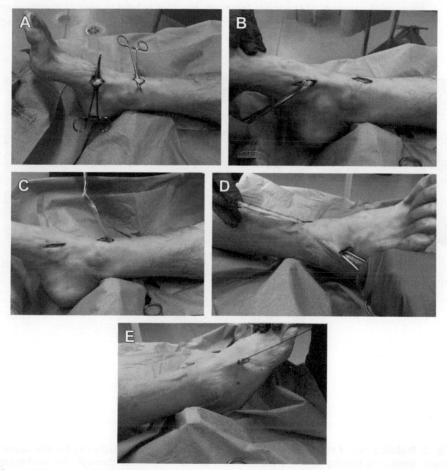

Fig. 2. Complete tibialis anterior tendon transfer. The tendon is identified and isolated through incisions 1 and 2 (*A*). The tendon is released completely from its insertion point through incision 1 (*B*) and drawn out through the anterior lower leg incision (incision 2; *C*). The end of the tendon is whipstitched and retrieved with the use of a hemostat from incision 3 underneath the extensor retinaculum (*D*, *E*).

foot incision. The tendon is then secured to the lateral cuneiform or the cuboid to appropriately balance the foot. Two methods of fixation exist.

- Interference screw (**Fig. 3**): A guidewire is placed from dorsal to plantar through the anchoring bone and retrieved through the plantar aspect of the foot. The tendon is sized, and the appropriate reamer for the interference screw is used over the previously placed guidewire. The tendon is passed through the prepared canal and out the plantar aspect of the foot. The foot is held in neutral dorsiflexion with slight eversion while appropriate physiologic tension is placed on the tendon. The interference screw is advanced from dorsal to plantar, securing the tendon. The suture is cut flush with the plantar aspect of the foot.
- Tendon anchor (**Fig. 4**): A tendon anchor of the surgeon's choice is placed from dorsal to plantar into the anchoring bone. The suture attached to the anchor is used to secure the tendon to the bone using a suture technique of the surgeon's choice. Excess tendon must be trimmed before suturing. To ensure that the appropriate amount of tendon is trimmed, the foot is held in neutral dorsiflexion with slight eversion, appropriate physiologic tension is placed on the tendon, and the tendon is trimmed accordingly.

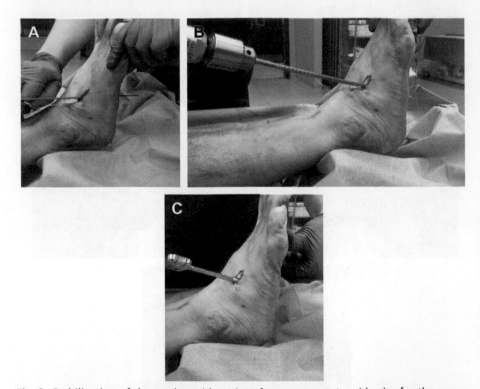

Fig. 3. Stabilization of the tendon with an interference screw. A guidewire for the appropriate sized interference screw is placed from dorsal to plantar through the anchoring bone exiting the plantar foot (*A*). This technique shows stabilization into the lateral cuneiform. The corresponding reamer is used over the guidewire (*B*), and the tendon is passed through the prepared hole exiting the plantar foot. With the foot dorsiflexed and slightly everted, the tendon is appropriately tensioned and the interference screw is advanced from dorsal to plantar, securing the tendon into the cuneiform (*C*).

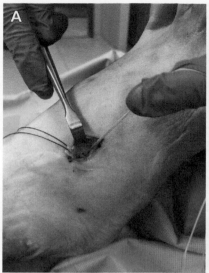
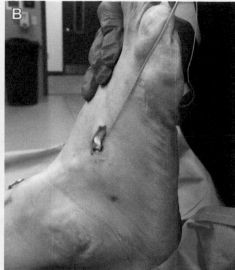

Fig. 4. Stabilization of the tendon with an anchor. An appropriately sized tendon anchor is inserted into the anchoring bone from dorsal to plantar (*A*). This technique shows stabilization into the lateral cuneiform. After the tendon is trimmed appropriately, the suture from the anchor is used to secure the tendon to the bone (*B*). The foot is held in dorsiflexion with slight eversion and appropriate tension is placed on the tendon.

Split tibialis anterior tendon transfer

Similar to the complete tibialis anterior tendon transfer described, the tendon is identified in the dorsal–medial foot and anterior leg incisions (**Fig. 5**). Once the tendon is identified within the anterior leg (incision 2), the tibialis anterior tendon is incised in a linear fashion. Umbilical tape is thread through the split and retrieved with the use of a tendon passer from proximal to distal, exiting through the medial foot incision (incision 1). This maneuver splits the tendon in half longitudinally. The lateral fibers of the tibialis anterior are released from the insertion point, and the freed portion of the tendon is pulled gently out of the anterior leg incision. The remainder of the procedure mirrors that of the tibialis anterior tendon transfer, as described.

Surgical Closure

After thorough irrigation of the surgical incisions, layered closure is performed in the standard fashion.

Immediate Postoperative Care

Patients are placed in a postoperative splint, with care taken to ensure that the foot is dorsiflexed in a neutral position with slight eversion. Strict non–weight-bearing status is initiated and maintained for 6 weeks. Suture removal occurs between 2 and 3 weeks, based on the extent of edema and incision coaptation.

REHABILITATION AND RECOVERY

Non–weight-bearing begins immediately after surgery. A postoperative splint is applied to maintain the desired foot position and adjusted accordingly over the course of 6 weeks. The patient is then graduated to a controlled ankle motion boot with progressive weight bearing. At this juncture, rehabilitation is initiated. Therapy focuses on tibialis

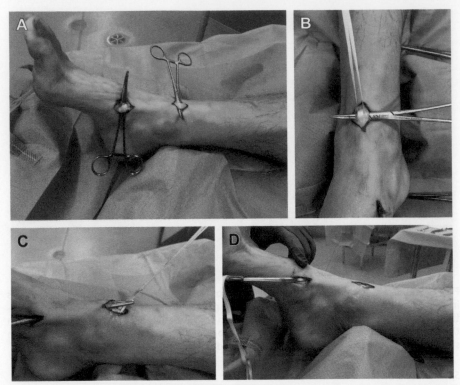

Fig. 5. Split tibialis anterior tendon transfer. The tendon is identified and isolated through incisions 1 and 2 (*A*). The tendon is splint longitudinally within incision 2, and umbilical tape is thread through the split (*B*). A hemostat is inserted into the tendon sheath through incision 1 to retrieve the umbilical tape (*C*). As the tape is pulled distally, the tendon is split longitudinally to its insertion point (*D*). The lateral half of the tendon is then released from its insertion point and drawn through the anterior lower leg incision (incision 3; *E*). The end of the tendon is whipstitched and retrieved with the use of a hemostat from incision 3 underneath the extensor retinaculum (*F, G*).

anterior muscle retraining, gait training, and progressive strengthening. The in-phase transfer of the tibialis anterior is beneficial to recovery, because the original function of the tendon is preserved and functional gains can be more rapidly achieved. Return to full activity depends on functional improvements with rehabilitation. Complete functional recovery is typically achieved within three to five months. The rehabilitation course should be altered in accordance with the performance of concomitant procedures. If non–weight-bearing is anticipated beyond six weeks, it is still recommended that the patient begin physical therapy with active, open chain motion, and muscle training.

COMPLICATIONS

Morbidity associated with this procedure is relatively low; however, complications can occur. **Table 3** provides a list of potential complications.

CLINICAL RESULTS IN THE LITERATURE

Tibialis anterior tendon transfers are used to address soft tissue imbalances and instabilities. With nonreducible deformities, however, bony procedures are often needed to

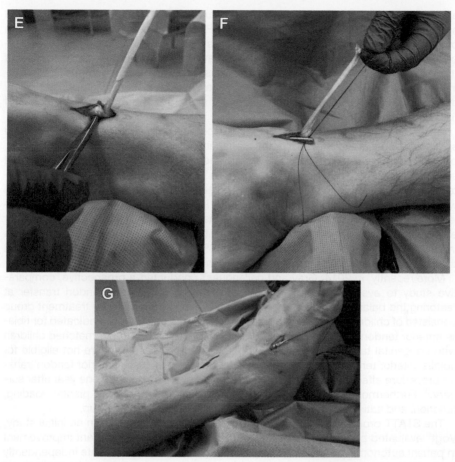

Fig. 5. (*continued*).

Table 3	
Complications associated with tibialis anterior tendon transfer	
Complication	**Iatrogenic Factors**
Infection	Transfer of the tendon too far laterally[12] or use of a split
Overcorrection	transfer over a full transfer[16]
Undercorrection	Inappropriate or absence of necessary concomitant procedures
Instability	Unopposed extensor hallucas longus and peroneus longus
Muscle necrosis	
Rupture of tendon transfer	
Damage to neurovascular structures[12,19]	
Transient tenosynovitis[12,13]	
Cocked-up hallux[20]	

Data from Refs.[12,13,16,19,20]

address the structural abnormalities. Consequently, the procedure is often tailored specifically to the deformity and the patient. Further complicating the interpretation of the results, numerous variations of the tibialis anterior tendon transfer have been reported since its initial introduction. Surgeons have described subcutaneous transfer of the tibialis anterior,[10] transfer through a 2-incision approach,[21] transfer through a 3-incision approach,[21] and split transfer.[22] The tendon can be rerouted above or below the extensor retinaculum[23] with variable sites of fixation and methods of fixation.[9,10,14,24,25]

Given the similar indications for the transfer of the tibialis anterior, the complete and split procedures are often used for the management of the same or similar conditions, both providing consistent results. Even so, the two procedures are often examined separately. In 2009, Thompson and colleagues[10] sought to determine whether subcutaneous tibialis anterior tendon transfer effectively treats recurrent clubfoot and whether the presence of structural deformities influenced the outcomes. Using a subjective rating system, the study confirmed that the tibialis anterior tendon transfer effectively restores muscle balance in recurrent clubfeet with resultant improvements in function. Balance was restored in 87% to 88% of patients with data to suggest that the tibialis anterior tendon transfer may prevent secondary osseous alteration.[10]

More recently, in 2014, Gray and colleagues[9] conducted a prospective, comparative study to evaluate the effectiveness of the tibialis anterior tendon transfer at restoring the balance between eversion and inversion strength. The treatment group consisted of children with idiopathic congenital talipes equinovarus indicated for tibialis anterior tendon transfer, and the control group consisted of age-matched children with congenital talipes equinovarus who, after Ponseti casting, were not eligible for tibialis anterior tendon transfer. The study found that the tibialis anterior tendon transfer procedure effectively restored the inversion to eversion balance one year after surgery.[9] Furthermore, the treatment group demonstrated similar plantar loading, function, and satisfaction outcomes compared with the control group.

The STATT procedure has also demonstrated favorable results. In an initial study, Vogt[6] evaluated patient outcomes after STATT and found a significant improvement in patient autonomy, demonstrated by an improved ability to ambulate independently and a decreased need to wear orthopedic shoes and orthoses, as well as an increased ability to wear normal shoes. The authors concluded that the procedure is safe and yields good results with minimal complications.[6] In 2011, Vogt and colleagues[7] retrospectively evaluated the functional results associated with the STATT procedure. Patients with spastic equinovarus deformity that were treated with the STATT procedure were asked to complete a questionnaire. The results showed a strong relationship between the preservation of deep foot sensitivity and the level of functional autonomy.[7]

There are a select number of comparative investigations evaluating the complete transfer of the tibialis anterior and the STATT. In 1998, Hui and colleagues[26] used a cadaveric model to determine if one procedure was more efficacious than the other. Despite the variation in techniques, the two procedures achieved similar maximum dorsiflexion. Also using a cadaver model, Knutsen and colleagues[21] found that the 2-incision complete transfer, the 3-incision complete transfer, and the split transfer produced varying forefoot pronation and hindfoot valgus motion. Notably, the 3-incision complete transfer and the split transfer demonstrated greater forefoot pronation compared with the 2-incision complete transfer.[21] Although both studies provide interesting insight, their cadaveric nature limits clinical translation. A cadaveric model cannot take into account the relative imbalance between the invertors and evertors to determine the appropriate amount of correction.

In 2001, Kuo and colleagues[17] conducted an in vivo study to compare the results of the complete transfer of the tibialis anterior tendon with the STATT in patients with residual dynamic clubfoot deformity. Both techniques provided satisfactory correction of the deformity. Employing Garceau's criteria, the two groups showed similar results. Moreover, both groups demonstrated a similar increase in dorsiflexion, plantar flexion, eversion, and motion at the tibiotalar joint. However, the STATT group demonstrated better preservation of inversion. With regard to muscle strength, both groups demonstrated similar increases in plantar flexion strength and eversion strength. There was no improvement in dorsiflexion strength for either group. The radiographic analysis revealed similar improvements in the anteroposterior talo-first metatarsal angle, the lateral talo-first metatarsal angle, and the overlap ratio. No significant correction in the lateral first to fifth metatarsal angle was observed for either group.[17]

Regardless of the operative approach, complete or STATT, the surgeon must decide whether to transfer the tendon above or below the extensor retinaculum. Ezra and colleagues[23] advocate the transfer of the tendon above the extensor retinaculum. Although this technique is thought to address the deformity appropriately, investigators have theorized that transferring the tendon underneath the retinaculum will decrease the incidence of postoperative transient tendonitis as well as the prominence of the tendon along the anterior leg. For these reasons, the authors advocate the transfer of the tendon beneath the extensor retinaculum.

Throughout the literature, a number of surgeons have described various sites for tibialis anterior tendon stabilization, including the lateral cuneiform, cuboid, and base of the fifth metatarsal. The evidence suggests that the ideal insertion site of the tibialis anterior tendon is onto the third metatarsal axis and the fourth metatarsal axis for the total tendon transfer and the split tendon transfer, respectively.[26] These sites were identified based on the maximum motion achieved at the foot and ankle, when the tendon was anchored and tension was applied. The same protocol was repeated serially from the second through the fifth metatarsals. As with many operative procedures, however, surgeon preference and the extent of deformity correction necessary often dictate insertion site selection.

Over the last 70 years, multiple methods of fixation have become available. Trephine plugs,[24] stabilization with a suture button and without osseous fixation,[9,10] interference screws,[22] bone anchors[25] and suture into the peroneus brevis[14] have proved viable. In a strength comparison, however, interference screws demonstrated superior strength compared with bone anchors for fixation during an STATT procedure.[25]

Despite a growing body of evidence, there is insufficient evidence to advocate one procedure over another. This is attributable in part to isolated examination of each procedure as opposed to direct comparisons, and in part to slight variations in the techniques and patient populations, which preclude direct comparisons. Be that as it may, many surgeons have described the STATT procedure as more reliable[12,17] and have recognized the STATT procedure for achieving adequate inversion to eversion muscle balance, presumably reducing the incidence of overcorrection.[16]

SUMMARY

With dynamic deformity correction, restoration of muscle balance can achieve improvements in function and prevent deformity progression. Both the complete transfer and STATT procedures result in similar improvements in ankle and foot range of motion and muscle function. However, the split transfer resulted in better preservation of the inversion motion. Kuo and colleagues[17] recognize that both procedures "are an excellent method of correcting residual dynamic clubfoot deformity," but prefer the split technique under the premise that it is less likely to result in overcorrection. However, considering the results, surgeon preference and patient presentation should dictate procedure selection.

REFERENCES

1. Garceau GJ. Anterior tibial tendon transposition in recurrent congenital clubfoot. J Bone Joint Surg Am 1940;22:932–6. Available at: http://jbjs.org/content/22/4/932.
2. Garceau GJ, Palmer RM. Transfer of the anterior tibial tendon for recurrent club foot. A long-term follow-up. J Bone Joint Surg Am 1967;49:207–31. Available at: http://jbjs.org/content/49/2/207.abstract.
3. Ponseti IV, Campos J. The classic: observations on pathogenesis and treatment of congenital clubfoot. 1972. Clin Orthop Relat Res 2009;467:1124–32. Available at: http://www.ncbi.nlm.nih.gov/pmc/articles/PMC2664437/.
4. Ponseti IV, Smoley EN. The classic: congenital club foot: the results of treatment. 1963. Clin Orthop Relat Res 2009;467:1133–45. Available at: http://www.ncbi.nlm.nih.gov/pmc/articles/PMC2664436/.
5. Hoffer MM, Reiswig JA, Garrett AM, et al. The split anterior tibial tendon transfer in the treatment of spastic varus hindfoot of childhood. Orthop Clin North Am 1974;5:31–8. Available at: http://www.ncbi.nlm.nih.gov/pubmed/4809542.
6. Vogt JC. Split anterior tibial transfer for spastic equinovarus foot deformity: retrospective study of 73 operated feet. J Foot Ankle Surg 1998;37:2–7 [discussion: 78]. Available at: http://www.sciencedirect.com/science/article/pii/S1067251698800033.
7. Vogt JC, Bach G, Cantini B, et al. Split anterior tibial tendon transfer for varus equinus spastic foot deformity initial clinical findings correlate with functional results: a series of 132 operated feet. Foot Ankle Surg 2011;17:178–81. Available at: http://www.footanklesurgery-journal.com/article/S1268-7731(10)00075-5/abstract.
8. Hoffer MM, Barakat G, Koffman M. 10-year follow-up of split anterior tibial tendon transfer in cerebral palsied patients with spastic equinovarus deformity. J Pediatr Orthop 1985;5:432–4. Available at: http://journals.lww.com/pedorthopaedics/Abstract/1985/07000/10_Year_Follow_up_of_Split_Anterior_Tibial_Tendon.8.aspx.
9. Gray K, Burns J, Little D, et al. Is tibialis anterior tendon transfer effective for recurrent clubfoot? Clin Orthop Relat Res 2014;472:750–8. Available at: http://www.ncbi.nlm.nih.gov/pmc/articles/PMC3890208/.
10. Thompson GH, Hoyen HA, Barthel T. Tibialis anterior tendon transfer after clubfoot surgery. Clin Orthop Relat Res 2009;467:1306–13. Available at: http://www.ncbi.nlm.nih.gov/pmc/articles/PMC2664443/.
11. Lampasi M, Bettuzzi C, Palmonari M, et al. Transfer of the tendon of tibialis anterior in relapsed congenital clubfoot: long-term results in 38 feet. J Bone Joint Surg Br 2010;92:277–83. Available at: http://www.bjj.boneandjoint.org.uk/content/92-B/2/277.long.
12. Banks AS, Downey MS, Martin DE, et al. Principles of muscle-tendon surgery and tendon transfers. In: Reilly CM, editor. McGlamry's comprehensive textbook of foot and ankle surgery. 3rd edition. Philadelphia: Lippincott Williams & Wilkins; 2001. p. 1523–66.
13. Johnson CH. Tendon transfers. In: Chang TJ, editor. Master techniques in podiatric surgery: the foot and ankle. Philadelphia: Lippincott Williams & Wilkins; 2004. p. 249–63.

14. Dreher T, Wenz W. Tendon transfers for the balancing of hind and mid-foot deformities in adults and children. Tech Foot Ankle Surg 2009;8:178–89. Available at: http://journals.lww.com/techfootankle/Abstract/2009/12000/Tendon_Transfers_for_the_Balancing_of_Hind_and.6.aspx.

15. Atesalp S, Bek D, Demiralp B, et al. Correction of residual dynamic varus deformity using the tibialis anterior tendon. J Bone Joint Surg Br 2006;88(sup 1):23–4. Available at: http://www.bjjprocs.boneandjoint.org.uk/content/88-B/SUPP_I/23.6.abstract.

16. Vlachou M, Dimitriadis D. Split tendon transfers for the correction of spastic varus foot deformity: a case series study. J Foot Ankle Res 2010;28:3. Available at: http://www.jfootankleres.com/content/3/1/28.

17. Kuo KN, Hennigan SP, Hastings ME. Anterior tibial tendon transfer in residual dynamic clubfoot deformity. J Pediatr Orthop 2001;21:35–41. Available at: http://journals.lww.com/pedorthopaedics/Abstract/2001/01000/Anterior_Tibial_Tendon_Transfer_in_Residual.9.aspx.

18. Keenan MA. The management of spastic equinovarus deformity following stroke and head injury. Foot Ankle Clin 2011;16:499–514. Available at: http://www.sciencedirect.com/science/article/pii/S1083751511000532.

19. Radler C, Gourdine-Shaw MC, Herzenberg JE. Nerve structures at risk in the plantar side of the foot during anterior tibial tendon transfer: a cadaver study. J Bone Joint Surg Am 2012;94:349–55. Available at: http://jbjs.org/content/94/4/349.long.

20. Singer M, Fripp AT. Tibialis anterior transfer in congenital club foot. J Bone Joint Surg Br 1958;40-B:252–5. Available at: http://www.bjj.boneandjoint.org.uk/content/40-B/2/252.long.

21. Knutsen AR, Avoian T, Sangiorgio SN, et al. How do different anterior tibial tendon transfer techniques influence forefoot and hindfoot motion? Clin Orthop Relat Res 2015;473:1737–43. Available at: http://link.springer.com/article/10.1007%2Fs11999-014-4057-0.

22. Wu KW, Huang S, Kuo KN, et al. The use of bioabsorbable screw in a split anterior tibial tendon transfer: a preliminary result. J Pediatr Orthop B 2009;18:69–72. Available at: http://journals.lww.com/jpo-b/Abstract/2009/03000/The_use_of_bioabsorbable_screw_in_a_split_anterior.4.aspx.

23. Ezra E, Hayek S, Gilai AN, et al. Tibialis anterior tendon transfer for residual dynamic supination deformity in treated club feet. J Pediatr Orthop B 2000;9:207–11. Available at: http://journals.lww.com/jpo-b/Abstract/2000/06000/Tibialis_Anterior_Tendon_Transfer_for_Residual.12.aspx.

24. Barnes MJ, Herring JA. Combined split anterior tibial-tendon transfer and intra-muscular lengthening of the posterior tibial tendon. Results in patients who have a varus deformity of the foot due to spastic cerebral palsy. J Bone Joint Surg Am 1991;73:734–8. Available at: http://jbjs.org/content/73/5/734.long.

25. Núñez-Pereira S, Pacha-Vicente D, Llusá-Pérez M, et al. Tendon transfer fixation in the foot and ankle: a biomechanical study. Foot Ankle Int 2009;30:1207–11. Available at: http://fai.sagepub.com/content/30/12/1207.short.

26. Hui JH, Goh JCH, Lee EH. Biomechanical study of tibialis anterior tendon transfer. Clin Orthop Relat Res 1998;349:249–55. Available at: http://journals.lww.com/corr/Abstract/1998/04000/Biomechanical_Study_of_Tibialis_Anterior_Tendon.31.aspx.

Jones Tendon Transfer

Richard Derner, DPM, FACFAS[a,b,]*, Jeffrey Holmes, DPM[c]

KEYWORDS

- Jones tendon transfer • Cavus foot • Claw hallux • Hallux malleus

KEY POINTS

- Jones tendon transfer or Jones tenosuspension is a tendon transfer performed to remove the deforming force for hallux malleus deformity. It is most often performed with interphalangeal joint (IPJ) fusion of the hallux.
- Indications include hallux malleus, in conjunction with cavus foot, caused most commonly by progressive peripheral neuropathy.
- The goal of this tendon transfer is not to elevate the first metatarsal. The intact peroneus longus (PL) tendon, which has maintained the plantar flexed position of the first metatarsal, prevents significant elevation alone by this tendon transfer.
- The complications associated with this procedure are minimal and related either to rupture of the tendon or stress fracture to the first metatarsal as a result of the hole made for the tendon transfer.

INTRODUCTION

Sir Robert Jones first described the Jones tendon transfer, or Jones tenosuspension, in 1916.[1] An orthopedic surgeon in the British military, Jones was also credited with the first description of a transverse fracture at the metaphyseal/diaphyseal junction at the base of the fifth metatarsal, the Jones fracture. In his 1916 article, Jones described a surgical procedure for the treatment of clawfoot with a coexisting clawed hallux.[2]

Jones described 5 degrees of deformity for the treatment of the clawfoot. The first degree develops in childhood. It is not associated with any significant deformity, and patients have more subjective complaints, such as clumsiness, often tripping over their feet with activity. A patient's physical examination can reveal a tight heel cord, but no structural deformity is observed. Stretching is the only treatment necessary to resolve this problem. The second degree of clawfoot is described as follows: flexible in nature with a contracture of the plantar fascia, Achilles tendon, and contracture of the hallux. This type of clawfoot deformity required transfer of the extensor hallucis longus (EHL)

Disclosure: No funding or conflict of interest.
[a] Associated Foot & Ankle Centers of Northern Virginia, 1721 Financial Loop, Lake Ridge, VA 22192, USA; [b] Inova Fairfax Medical Campus, 3300 Gallows Road, Falls Church, VA 22042-3300, USA; [c] Inova Fairfax Medical Campus, PGY-3, 3300 Gallows Road, Original Building, Falls Church, VA 22042-3300, USA
* Corresponding author. American College of Foot and Ankle Surgeons, 1721 Financial Loop, Woodbridge, VA 22192.
E-mail address: Richd87@mac.com

Clin Podiatr Med Surg 33 (2016) 55–62
http://dx.doi.org/10.1016/j.cpm.2015.06.004
0891-8422/16/$ – see front matter © 2016 Elsevier Inc. All rights reserved.

tendon. The Jones tendon transfer was described as a transfer of the EHL from its insertion, through the neck of the first metatarsal and tied on itself. Jones combined this tendon transfer with an incision of the plantar fascia.[2] Over the years, the indications have remained similar to Jones' original description in the literature. The IPJ fusion of the hallux was added to the description with the tendon transfer in recent literature.

The third degree of the clawfoot described by Jones was a rigid contracture of the lesser digits at the metatarsophalangeal joint (MPJ) level as well as the hallux. Tendon transfer was not performed in the later stages due to the fixed deformity of the lesser toes. The forth and fifth degrees were described as fixed in nature and had the same contracture as noted by the third degree but with an equinovarus deformity. In the most severe cases, fifth degree, Jones recommended a distal amputation removing all the toes as well as metatarsal heads.[2]

INDICATION/ETIOLOGY

The Jones tendon transfer is performed for the treatment of the clawed hallux or hallux malleus deformity. Typically, this tendon transfer is performed in combination with a hallux IPJ fusion. A clawed hallux is defined as extension of the first MPJ and flexion of the IPJ. The deformity is attributed to muscular imbalances that include the intrinsic musculature, the *flexor hallucis longus* (FHL) tendon, the EHL tendon, and the PL tendon.[3] The cause of this imbalance has yet to be quantitatively described. Several studies have implicated that the 3 extrinsic muscles acting on the hallux are thought to be the main deforming forces, but the intrinsic muscles may have a more significant role than previously thought.[1,4] Olson and colleagues,[4] in 2003, looked at the 3 extrinsic muscles acting on the hallux in a cadaveric study. The investigators concluded the main attribute that led to plantar flexion of the first metatarsal that leads to increased pressure under the first metatarsal head is due overpowering of the PL tendon. Overpowering of the EHL resulted in the excessive extension deformity of the MPJ and the pull of the FHL led to the largest deformity of the IPJ, which caused increase pressure under the hallux. Giannini and colleagues,[1] in 1985, concluded the etiology of the hallux claw toe was a cause of muscular imbalances but the FHL and EHL are not the main factors and might contribute and aggravate the deformity.[1]

The closed kinetic chain function of the intrinsic muscles is to stabilize the hallux to the ground at the MPJ. Weakness or overpowering of the intrinsic muscles by the extrinsic muscles is the cause of hallux malleus deformity, resulting in the contracture at the MPJ and flexion deformity at the IPJ.

There are 2 specific categories that result in the muscular imbalance causing claw toe deformity. The etiology can be either neurologic or idiopathic. Idiopathic refers to an unspecified cause of the deformity. The neurologic group can be further divided into either a result from an upper motor neuron disease (spastic) or lower motor neuron disease (flaccid). Charcot-Marie-Tooth (CMT), poliomyelitis, Roussy-Lévy syndrome, and Friedreich ataxia are the most common lower motor neuron diseases causing disorders of the foot and lower extremities. CMT is the best-studied and most common disorder causing a cavus deformity. Approximately 90% of patients with CMT present with a cavus foot deformity.[5] A study by Palma and colleagues,[6] in 21 subjects treated with a Jones procedure for clawed hallux, reported that 6 had poliomyelitis, 3 had cerebral palsy, 3 had spina bifida, 2 had unknown neurologic disease, and 7 were idiopathic cavus feet. A study by Kadel and colleagues,[7] however, reported a large dominance in CMT compared with other patient populations when seeing a clawed hallux. The mechanism that leads to the hallux claw toe is recruitment of the EHL and extensor digitorum longus as accessory dorsiflexors, to balance the weakness of the tibialis anterior.[5]

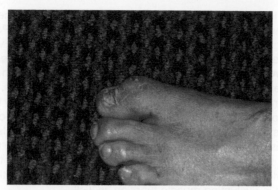

Fig. 1. Callosity to dorsal IPJ of the hallux.

CLINICAL EVALUATION

The main complaints caused by the hallux malleus deformity are pain, preulcer lesions/active ulcers, poor fitting shoe gear, and cosmesis. Because hallux malleus is often a result of a neurologic disease, a thorough history and physical are imperative. A neurologic evaluation of the patient may impart a great deal during the physical examination. Muscle strength evaluation on both extremities is important when considering the Jones tendon transfer. Special attention should be directed to the hallux MTP, IPJs, and the 3 extrinsic muscles of the hallux.

Dermatologically, callosities and ulcers can be seen, denoting increase pressure. It is not unusual to find ulcers in patients with neuropathy as a result of the hallux malleus deformity. It is best if the ulcers can be resolved prior to surgery, if possible. Classically, there are lesions dorsally at the IPJ (**Figs. 1** and **2**) and plantarly either at the distal aspect of the hallux or sub–first metatarsal head.

When examining the range of motion to the hallux, it is important to evaluate the first ray completely, including the first metatarsal-cuneiform joint, first MPJ, and hallux IPJ. A fixed plantar flexed position first ray necessitates a dorsiflexory wedge osteotomy of the first metatarsal to resolve the plantar pressure under the first MPJ joint. If a Jones procedure alone or in combination with an IPJ fusion is used to correct a clawed hallux with a fixed plantar flexed first ray, there will be only mild improvement to the plantar pressure beneath the first metatarsal head.

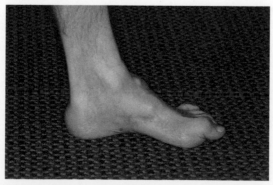

Fig. 2. Clawfoot with coexisting clawed hallux.

Evaluation of the first MPJ is also critical. If there is arthrosis to the first MPJ, care must be given when considering both a fusion of the first MPJ and IPJ. This is a challenging problem, and poor positioning results in continued pain. Even with perfect placement of these 2 joint fusions, problems may occur for the patient.

Radiographic evaluation consisting of weight-bearing images of the foot and ankle are assessed carefully to further evaluate the deformity to the great toe. Anteroposterior and lateral radiographs are taken at a minimum but oblique views may help evaluate for any arthrosis or other deformities. Determining the severity of the cavus deformity, arthrosis of the first ray, and great toe complex is critical in treatment planning. Previous surgeries and present deformities all are examined with preoperative radiographs.

Other imaging modalities, such as MRI, may give insight as to tendon location, especially if previous surgery has been performed. Nerve conduction studies may be ordered to aid in evaluating muscle function as well.

JONES TENDON TRANSFER SURGERY

The goal of the Jones tendon transfer is to remove the deforming force at the first MPJ and IPJ. This tendon transfer procedure was never intended to aid in elevation of the first ray. Classically, a transferred tendon loses a grade of muscle strength once relocated. Therefore, the intact strong PL tendon, which plantar flexes the first ray, does not yield to this now much weaker EHL tendon. By understanding the components causing the deformity, removing the deforming tendon has successful reproducible results.

The surgical procedure is almost never performed alone and most often accomplished in conjunction with a hallux IPJ fusion. In more severe foot deformities, many other procedures are performed at the same operative setting. The incision is made medial to the long extensor tendon to the hallux and then in a lazy-S fashion brought across the hallux IPJ laterally and completed distal laterally short of the nail root of the hallux nail plate (Fig. 3). The tendon is then transected distally and freed up proximal to the MPJ. All procedures, including the IPJ fusion and dorsiflexory wedge osteotomy (Fig. 4) to the first metatarsal, are completed prior to completing the tendon transfer. A drill hole is made through the neck of the metatarsal oriented transversely from medial to lateral. This needs to be big enough to allow for transfer of the tendon but not too big, which could result in a stress riser. The tendon is the transferred from lateral to medial and tied on itself dorsally under physiologic tension with nonabsorbable suture (Figs. 5 and 6). In long-standing deformities, a dorsal capsulotomy at the first MPJ may be required to allow for structural realignment of the hallux.

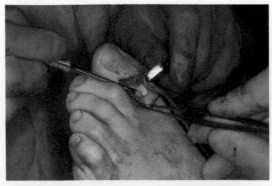

Fig. 3. Dissection of the IPJ with deattachment of the EHL tendon.

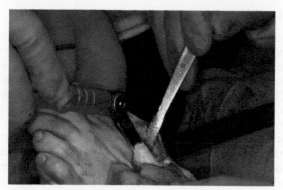

Fig. 4. Dorsiflexory wedge osteotomy to the first metatarsal.

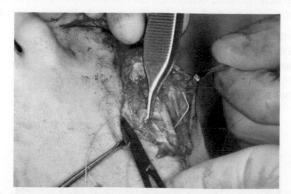

Fig. 5. The EHL being pulled through a drill hole lateral to medial and tied on itself.

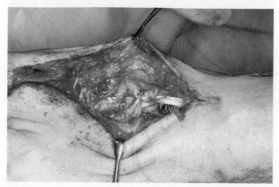

Fig. 6. The EHL has been sutured with nonabsorbable suture. Also showing a finished dorsi-flexory wedge osteotomy.

ADJUNCT PROCEDURES

The Jones procedure is now commonly performed in conjunction with an IPJ arthrodesis. The combined procedure is widely accepted to allow for realignment of the first MPJ and stabilize the hallux. Without antagonistic pull against the FHL, a mallet toe is the result, if fusion of the IPJ were not performed. An alternative to the modified Jones is a tenodesis of the IPJ by attaching the stump of the EHL to the proximal phalanx. This technique is indicated particularly in children in whom an arthrodesis may damage the physis of the distal phalanx.

With a fixed plantar flexed first ray deformity, a dorsiflexory wedge osteotomy must be performed to elevate the first metatarsal. The Jones tendon transfer does not allow for any significant dorsiflexion of the first metatarsal. The osteotomy needs to be performed first, followed by the tendon transfer. The fixation and technique is again surgeon preference, but the authors' is single screw fixation for this first metatarsal osteotomy. In children, care must be taken to protect the proximal physis of the first metatarsal.

There are many other concomitant procedures that may be implemented with the Jones tendon transfer. Also a hindfoot, midfoot, or forefoot deformity or a combination (flexible or fixed) may be seen in which osseous and soft tissue work needs to be performed. It is rare that an isolated hallux claw toe is seen that makes the history and physical that much more important when evaluating this patient population (**Figs. 7** and **8**).

- Concomitant procedures
  - ○ Tibialis anterior transfer (complete)
    - ▪ Split tibialis anterior tendon transfer
    - ▪ Dorsiflexory wedge osteotomy of the first metatarsal
  - ○ Plantar fascia release (Steindler stripping)

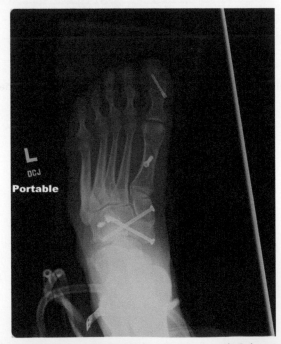

Fig. 7. Cavus foot reconstruction postoperative radiograph with Cole osteotomy, PT tendon transfer, dorsiflexory wedge osteotomy, and a modified Jones procedure.

- Triple arthrodesis, medial double arthrodesis
- Tarsal wedge osteotomy, such as a Cole.
- Calcaneal osteotomy
  - Hibbs tendon transfer
  - Proximal interphalangeal joint arthrodesis of the lesser toes
- Posterior tibial tendon transfer
- FHL-to-EHL tendon transfer

POSTOPERATIVE MANAGEMENT

Postoperatively, patients are placed in a posterior splint for a few days. From that point, depending on the other procedures performed, a below-the-knee fiberglass cast is applied for approximately 4 weeks. Care must be taken not to allow patients to plantar flex or actively dorsiflex their foot prior to that time. Rupture of the tendon may result. Furthermore, weight bearing should be guarded at first, after approximately 4 weeks, to prevent fracture of the first metatarsal drill hole.

DISCUSSION

The Jones tendon transfer has been implemented for approximately 100 years. Over the years, the accepted procedure is the modified Jones tendon transfer where the IPJ is fused during the tendon transfer.

Döderlein and colleagues[8,9] presented an article in which 81 modified Jones tendon transfers were carried out. After a 42-month average follow-up, 36 feet regarded their results as excellent, 38 feet as satisfactory, and only 7 feet as unsatisfactory. The most common complication associated in this study was an elevated first ray. Of the 25 feet noted to have an elevated first ray, a PL-to–peroneus brevis (PB) tendon transfer was performed in 21 of those (84%). Due to the high incidence of an elevated first ray with a PL-to-PB tendon transfer, the investigators did not recommend this procedure. Palma and colleagues[6] reviewed 24 feet that underwent a modified Jones tendon transfer. Of the 24 feet, 13 cases showed good results, 6 cases were described as fair, and 5 cases with poor results. There were significantly better results in patients who had an underlying etiology of neuromuscular disease compared with patients with an idiopathic cavovarus deformity. A retrospective study by M'Bamali[10] showed the modified Jones procedure for correction of clawed hallux deformity demonstrated that tendon regeneration of the distal EHL stump was a contributing factor in the recurrence of the clawed hallux deformity.

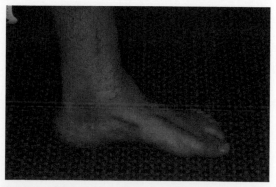

Fig. 8. Clinical examination of the patient after a modified Jones procedure was performed as well as a dorsiflexory wedge osteotomy with a rectus foot and no contracture seen to the first ray.

CONCLUSION

Hallux malleus is a deformity of the great toe attributed to muscular imbalance of various structures affecting the great toe. The Jones tendon transfer with the IPJ fusion is an effective procedure used for correcting the deformity. The modified Jones procedure is currently the preferred choice due to the previous complications of a hallux malleus arising from the original Jones procedure. There are many adjunct procedures that can also be used in the treatment of the cavus foot. These are often seen in conjunction with the hallux malleus deformity. A thorough evaluation of the patient must be performed prior to proceeding with the treatment of the contracted hallux.

REFERENCES

1. Giannini S, Girolammi M, Ceccarelli F, et al. Modified Jones operation in the treatment of pes cavovarus. Ital J Orthop Traumatol 1985;11:165–70.
2. Jones R. The soldier's foot and the treatment of common deformities of the foot, part II. Br Med J 1916;1:749–53.
3. Abousayed M, Kwon JY. Hallux claw toe. Foot Ankle Clin 2014;19(1):59–63.
4. Olson SL, Ledoux WR, Ching RP, et al. Muscular imbalances resulting in a clawed hallux. Foot Ankle Int 2003;24:477–85.
5. Faldini C. Surgical treatment of cavus foot in charcot-marie-tooth disease: a review of twenty-four cases: AAOS exhibit selection. J Bone Joint Surg Am 2015; 97(6):e30.
6. Palma LD, Colonna E, Travasi M. The modified Jones procedure for pes cavovarus with claw hallux. J Foot Ankle Surg 1997;36:279–83.
7. Kadel NJ, Donaldson-Fletcher EA, Hansen ST, et al. Alternative to the modified Jones procedure: outcomes of the flexor hallucis longus (FHL) tendon transfer procedure for correction of clawed hallux. Foot Ankle Int 2005;26:1021–6.
8. Döderlein L, Breusch S, Wenz W. Transfer of extensor hallucis longus tendon (modified Robert Jones procedure). J Orthop Traumatol 2000;8:273–84.
9. Döderlein L, Breusch S, Wenz W. Function after correction of a clawed great toe by a modified Robert Jones transfer. J Bone Joint Surg Br 2000;82(2):250–4.
10. M'Bamali EI. Results of the modified Robert Jones operation for clawed hallux. Br J Surg 1975;62:647–50.

Hibbs Tenosuspension

Sean T. Grambart, DPM

KEYWORDS

- Hibbs tenosuspension • Hibbs tendon transfer
- Extensor digitorum longus to midfoot • Charcot-Marie-Tooth • Extensor substitution

KEY POINTS

- The Hibbs tenosuspension is utilized to help correct contracture of the digits secondary to overpull of the extensor digitorum longus.
- Use of a Hibbs tenosuspension in isolation can only be effective if the digital contracture is fully reducible. If the contractures are semireducible or fixed, the digits should be corrected with proximal interphalangeal joint (PIPJ) arthrodesis.
- Transfer of the tendon should be into either the peroneus tertius or lateral cuneiform. The peroneus tertius needs to be large enough in diameter to support the transfer.

INTRODUCTION

The Hibbs tenosuspension is an underutilized procedure for the treatment of contracted digits. Reasons for this underutilization could be lack exposure to the procedure during surgical training, the fact that it is not commonly used as a single stand-alone procedure, or lack of literature on the procedure. A PubMed search using the terms Hibbs tenosuspension, Hibbs tendon transfer, and extensor digitorum longus to midfoot transfer yields a total of 3 results. The goal of this article is to describe the Hibbs tenosuspension to use for the contacted digits.

PATHOMECHANICS

The extensor digitorum longus (EDL) tendon is recruited to help with dorsiflexion in the presence of a weak tibialis anterior tendon and/or an overpowering Achilles tendon leading to forefoot equinus. As the tibialis anterior tendon is weakened, the recruitment of the EDL results in contracture of the proximal phalanx causing a retrograde force on the metatarsal head at the metatarsophalangeal joint that can lead to metatarsalgia and hammertoe or claw toe deformities (**Fig. 1**).

Conditions in which it is common to see include Charcot-Marie-Tooth disease and postpolio syndrome. Other conditions for which a Hibbs tenosuspension may be

Orthopedics, Carle Physician Group, 1802 South Mattis Avenue, Champaign, IL 61821, USA
E-mail address: Sean.grambart@carle.com

Clin Podiatr Med Surg 33 (2016) 63–69
http://dx.doi.org/10.1016/j.cpm.2015.07.001
0891-8422/16/$ – see front matter © 2016 Elsevier Inc. All rights reserved.

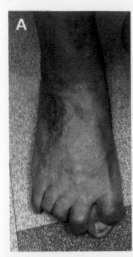
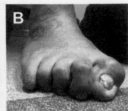
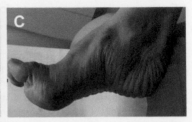

Fig. 1. (*A–C*) Preoperative appearance of toe deformities with example of extensor substitution.

beneficial include diabetes or rheumatoid arthritis in which the intrinsic musculature is weak, allowing the extrinsic EDL muscle to overpower the intrinsic muscles. In patients who have undergone a transmetatarsal amputation, the Hibbs tenosuspension is a nice adjunct procedure to prevent the overpull of the tibialis anterior tendon in order to prevent a varus deformity and lateral column overload.

There are relatively few contraindications for the procedure. The most obvious contraindication is a nonfunctioning or weak EDL. The author recommends digital arthrodesis with this procedure, so this can be done with reducible or nonreducible deformities. If the surgeon is doing the Hibbs tendon transfer as an isolated procedure, then the digital contractures must be fully reducible.

SURGICAL TECHNIQUE

The author prefers not to perform any toe work such as PIPJ arthrodesis until the EDL tendons are harvested in order to preserve the tension on the tendons to make the harvest easier. Once the tendons are harvested, then any osseous procedure on the toes or metatarsals can be performed.

The incision approach is through a curvilinear incision along the lateral–dorsal midfoot area typical starting at the base of the fourth metatarsal (**Fig. 2**). Care is made to identify branches of the intermediate dorsal cutaneous nerve. The EDL tendon sheath is incised, and the long extensor tendons are exposed (**Fig. 3**). If there is a peroneus tertius, it is identified proximal and lateral to the extensor tendons. The tertius must be substantial enough to hold the transfer of the tendons. The tendon should be at least 4 mm in diameter in order to facilitate the transfer. The presence or diameter of the tertius cannot be guaranteed, so be prepared to transfer the tendon to the lateral cuneiform, securing it in place with a biotenodesis screw.

All 4 extensor tendons are transected at the mid-metatarsal (**Fig. 4**). The lateral 2 tendons are stripped of their paratenon. Prior to the transfer, evaluate the angle of the lateral tendons. This should be a straight line of pull to the tertius or lateral cuneiform. If there is an oblique angle, this must be corrected to create a straight line of pull. This can often be done with taking a pair of Metzenbaum scissors and carefully sliding

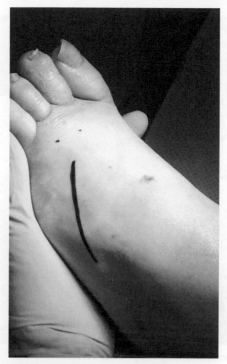

Fig. 2. Dorsolateral incision along the fourth metatarsal.

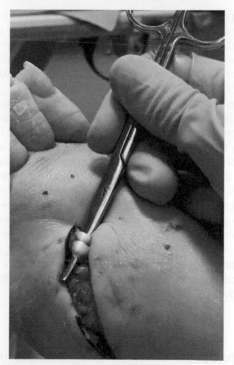

Fig. 3. Identification of the long extensor tendons.

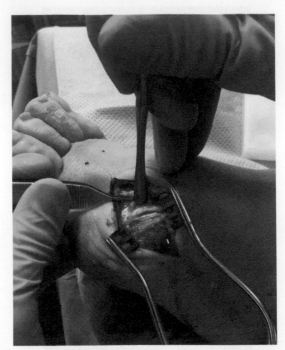

Fig. 4. Isolation of the extensor tendons prior to release.

it along the tendons proximally to release the sheath. In order to prevent accidental transection of the tendons, place the opening of the scissors perpendicular to the sheath. Transferring all 4 tendons will increase the potential of binding, so the tendons to the second and third metatarsal are trimmed more proximally (**Fig. 5**). The distal slips of the EDL tendons are transferred to the EDB tendons proximal to the metatarsophalangeal joints (MTPJs) (**Fig. 6**).

The peroneal tertius tendon is inspected to make sure it is adequate diameter to support a direct transfer (**Fig. 7**). The lateral 2 tendons are transferred under the tertius tendon (**Fig. 8**). The ankle is placed in neutral position, and the lateral 2 tendons are secured in place into the tertius tendon (**Fig. 9**). If there is not a tertius tendon or if the tendon is too small, transfer the lateral tendons into the lateral cuneiform and secure in place with a biotenodesis screw. Any continued extension deformities of the MTPJ should have been released prior with the initial bone work.

The postoperative course is typically based on the other procedures. In an isolated Hibbs procedure, the patient is kept nonweight-bearing in a splint at neutral position for 10 to 14 days. At this point, the patient may progress to a weight-bearing boot for 4 weeks. During this time, the boot can be removed when sitting, and range-of-motion exercises can be initiated. The patient sleeps in the boot or a splint positioned at neutral. At 6 weeks postoperatively, the patient can begin weight-bearing in shoes and slowly start to advance activities and shoe wear.

COMPLICATIONS

With careful dissection, most of the potential complications can be avoided. Numbness or dorsal nerve irritation is common for a short time during the

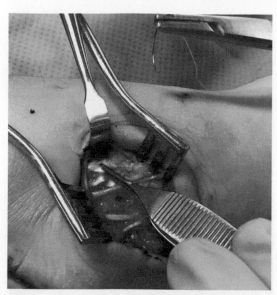

Fig. 5. Release of the long extensor tendon to the second toe.

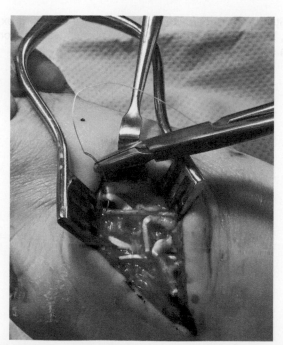

Fig. 6. Transfer of the long extensor tendon into the extensor digitorum brevis tendon.

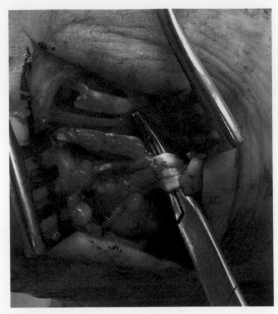

Fig. 7. Peroneus tertius greater than 4 mm diameter.

postoperative period, but can also be a long-term issue. Scar and binding of the tendon can lead to lack of function of the tendon transfer. However, the resolution of the digital contractures still results in a successful outcome even if the tendon does not work.

Results in the literature are scarce to say the least. In the author's experience, this is an ideal transfer, because it meets the criteria of taking away a deforming force and converting it to a stabilizing force (**Fig. 10**).

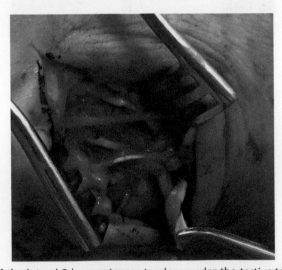

Fig. 8. Passing of the lateral 2 long extensor tendons under the tertius tendon.

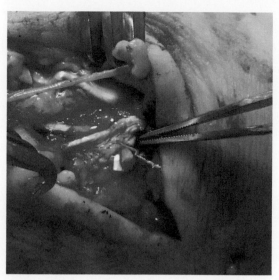

Fig. 9. Lateral 2 extensor tendons sutured into the tertius tendon.

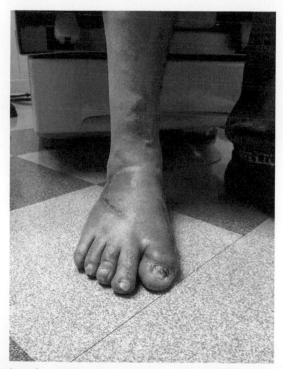

Fig. 10. Postoperative after Hibbs tenosuspension with arthrodesis of the lesser toes.

Tendon Transfers for Management of Digital and Lesser Metatarsophalangeal Joint Deformities

Michelle Butterworth, DPM*

KEYWORDS

- Flexor tendon transfer • Metatarsophalangeal joint • Hammertoe • Plantar plate
- Predislocation syndrome

KEY POINTS

- Biomechanical etiologies are a significant contributing factor to digital and metatarsophalangeal joint (MTPJ) deformities. They need to be identified and included in the evaluation and treatment plan.
- Tendon transfers for digital and MTPJ deformities are just one surgical option for correction. They are usually not stand-alone procedures, and typically, a combination of procedures is needed for full correction.
- A tendon should be transferred under physiologic tension. If the tension is too tight, stiffness will result. If not enough tension is utilized, recurrence of the deformity can result.
- The flexor digitorum longus tendon transfer has a high patient satisfaction rate when performed under the proper indications and with concomitant use of other procedures for full deformity correction.

 Video of Flexor Tendon Transfer for 2nd MTPJ instability accompanies this article at http://www.podiatric.theclinics.com/

INTRODUCTION

Digital and MTPJ deformities are common and unfortunately can be complex and challenging for the foot and ankle surgeon. Although these forefoot deformities may be thought of as just simple hammertoe deformities by some, the astute surgeon knows that their complex nature and contributing deforming forces dictate that each deformity be treated individually with an arsenal of treatment options available.

Disclosures: None.
Private Practice, Pee Dee Foot Center, 402 Nelson Boulevard, Suite 300, Kingstree, SC 29556, USA
* 308 Logan Street, Kingstree, SC 29556.
E-mail address: mbutter@ftc-i.net

Clin Podiatr Med Surg 33 (2016) 71–84
http://dx.doi.org/10.1016/j.cpm.2015.06.015
0891-8422/16/$ – see front matter © 2016 Elsevier Inc. All rights reserved.

Tendon transfers are just one option that can be added to the procedure selection for digital and MTPJ deformities, and they are typically not performed as stand-alone procedures. Usually, a combination of both osseous and soft tissue procedures is necessary to gain adequate correction of the deformity. A stepwise approach should be utilized to thoroughly evaluate the deformity, address all deforming forces, and devise an appropriate treatment regimen. The experienced surgeon realizes that these deformities are not the same and cannot be treated as such. What may work on one deformity may not work on another.

CAUSATIVE FACTORS

Biomechanical etiologies are the number one contributing factor to digital and MTPJ deformities; therefore, any force that creates increased and/or abnormal loading on the forefoot can cause digital derangement. First ray insufficiency can result from many entities, including, but not limited to medial column hypermobility and a shortened or elevated first metatarsal. This will increase lateral loading, and significant deformity of the lesser MTPJs and digits can result. In hallux abductovalgus deformity, lateral deviation of the hallux into the second toe can cause retrograde buckling at the second MTPJ and cause subluxation/dislocation (**Fig. 1**). Pes planovalgus, pes cavus, and equinus deformities can result in abnormal and increased forefoot loading and contribute to digital and MTPJ deformities. Structural deformities such as a long metatarsal can increase stress across the joint and contribute to lesser ray abnormalities. Of course trauma, both acute and repetitive, can always be a causative factor, and there are many systemic diseases that can contribute to joint degeneration and subluxation with resultant lesser digital and MTPJ deformity. Patients themselves can also be responsible for these deformities by wearing high-heeled shoes and increasing forefoot load.

Generally, digital deformities and malalignment at the MTPJ can be easily visualized, but in the early stages of lesser metatarsophalangeal joint pain and inflammation, there is usually lack of digital deformity or subluxation, and only symptomatology presents. This entity has been termed predislocation syndrome by Yu and colleagues.[1,2] The patient with predislocation syndrome usually has focal pain at the plantar aspect of the involved MTPJ. Pain is increased during ambulation, and patients usually state that they feel like they are walking on a lump. Localized edema, to varying degrees, is also typically present. Some patients mention a change in activity or start of a new athletic activity as a triggering factor for their pain and inflammation. Others may relate minor trauma such as a misstep or a twisting of their foot.

Subsequent progression of predislocation syndrome can ensue, especially if these entities are left untreated, and subluxation/dislocation of the MTPJ can result. Yu and colleagues[1,2] developed a classification system based on clinical findings:

Stage 1: mild edema plantarly, extreme tenderness of the joint, no anatomic malalignment
Stage 2: moderate edema with noticeable deviation of the digit clinically and radiographically; toe does not purchase ground
Stage 3: moderate edema, pronounced deviation

Stability of the lesser MTPJ is derived from the plantar plate, the collateral ligaments, and the intrinsic and extrinsic foot musculature. Static stabilization of the MTPJ is derived primarily from the plantar plate and collateral ligaments. Dynamic stabilization is provided by the intrinsic and extrinsic musculature. The ability of these muscles however, to stabilize the MTPJ is highly dependent on the integrity of the plantar plate.

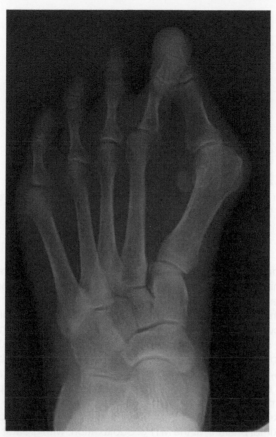

Fig. 1. Hypermobility has caused first ray insufficiency with resultant hallux abductovalgus deformity. The lateral deviation of the hallux, along with increased lateral load, has produced obvious subluxation of the second MTPJ.

The plantar plate is a distal attachment of the plantar fascia, and it has attachments to the deep transverse intermetatarsal ligament and the collateral ligaments. It is a fibrocartilagenous thickening of the MTPJ capsule plantarly, and it is firmly attached to the proximal phalanx (**Fig. 2**). The plantar plate also serves as the insertion for both the interossei and lumbrical tendons. Because the plantar plate provides a substantial static support for the lesser MTPJs, insufficiency involving tear, attenuation, or absence of this structure can result in significant sagittal plane instability and deformity. Through mechanical testing, Bhatia[3] found the plantar plate to be the main stabilizing force of the MTPJ, and the collateral ligaments were the second most powerful structures to stabilize the MTPJ.

The key developmental factor of subluxation of the MTPJ then is progressive inflammation about the joint with subsequent attenuation and rupture of the plantar plate and collateral ligaments. Therefore, as it has previously been stated, any structural deformity or biomechanical force that increases loading on the forefoot and results in inflammation of the periarticular structures can predispose the individual to weakening of the plantar plate and collateral ligaments and result in rupture and instability.

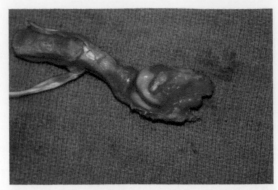

Fig. 2. The plantar plate is a fibrocartilagenous thickening of the plantar capsule and is firmly attached to the base of the proximal phalanx.

DIAGNOSIS

Diagnosis of predislocation syndrome can be challenging at times, and historically it has often been misdiagnosed as a neuroma. With increased awareness of the entity, however, physicians have become much more astute to the clinical findings and differentiation of other entities. A positive Thompson and Hamilton sign, or pain with pure vertical force across the MTPJ, is indicative of predislocation syndrome. The Lachman vertical stress test can also aid the physician in an accurate diagnosis and evaluation of plantar plate integrity. This clinical test is performed by stabilizing the metatarsal head with the thumb and index finger; then the contralateral hand is utilized to grip the dorsal and plantar aspect of the corresponding proximal phalangeal base. The digit is then manipulated upward with vertical pressure from the thumb plantarly. Care must be taken to ensure that this is truly a vertical upward force and not dorsiflexion of the proximal phalanx at the MTPJ. Subluxation, with greater than 50% dorsal displacement of the base of the proximal phalanx on the head of the metatarsal, is considered positive for plantar plate laxity (**Fig. 3**).

Imaging modalities can be a helpful, but typically clinical evaluation and standard radiographs are enough to diagnose and evaluate lesser digital and MTPJ deformities. Standard weight-bearing radiographs can be used to thoroughly evaluate the location

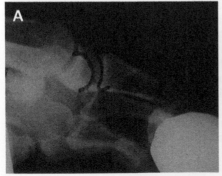
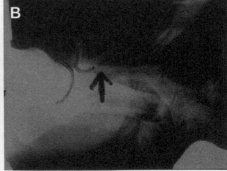

Fig. 3. Radiographic appearance of the Lachman vertical stress test showing rectus alignment of the proximal phalanx on the metatarsal head (*A*) then dorsal displacement of the proximal phalanx with applied vertical force indicating plantar plate laxity (*B*).

and specific type of ray deformity. The MTPJ can be examined for deviation, subluxation, and/or dislocation of the digit and decreased joint space or degenerative changes within the joint. There should also be evaluation of the metatarsal parabola and other structural abnormalities. Cortical thickening is often seen with the involved metatarsal and is a sign of metatarsal overload. One should also always evaluate for a possible stress fracture as part of the differential diagnosis.

Arthrography, ultrasound, and MRI have all been utilized and described as being beneficial in evaluating MTPJ integrity, in particular plantar plate rupture. Gregg and colleagues,[4] evaluated 25 plantar plates at surgery and found tears in 23 plates. They concluded that ultrasound was 96% sensitive compared with 87% sensitivity for MRI in detecting plantar plate tears in this group and that ultrasound was an inexpensive and safe alternative to MRI of the plantar plate.

CONSERVATIVE TREATMENT

Conservative treatment should always be attempted, and the goal is to reduce and/or eliminate pain and inflammation and prevent progression of the deformity. It is also important to identify the causative factors and address those when possible. Good biomechanical control with orthotics and appropriate shoe gear is always usually part of a successful treatment protocol. Stabilizing the digit and joint with appropriate strapping also typically helps with pain control and prevention of deformity progression. Nonsteroidal anti-inflammatory drugs and oral corticosteroids are the mainstay of treatment for pain and inflammation. Of course activity modification and physical therapy modalities are also beneficial for control of inflammation.

There is controversy regarding intra-articular steroid injections for this entity, but several authors have reported good success.[5–7] Mizel and Michaelson[7] reported a 70% success rate with 14 intra-articular steroid injections for nontraumatic synovitis, and Trepman and Yeo[6] reported a 93% success rate on 13 patients. Although proven to be beneficial by some authors, Reis and colleagues[8] reported 2 dislocations of the second toe after receiving an intra-articular steroid injection. Although repeated injections can cause joint distention and damage to the periarticular structures, many surgeons, including the author, feel that a phosphate, in controlled amounts, can be effectively and safely utilized for intra-articular injections into the lesser MTPJs. Several factors will influence the frequency of injections, however, including the type and quantity of corticosteroid utilized. The author does not support the use of intra-articular acetate injection for this entity. Also if an intra-articular injection is performed, one should stabilize the toe with appropriate strapping.

SURGICAL TREATMENT
Preoperative Planning

When conservative therapies fail to resolve pain, and inflammation or progression of the deformity ensues, surgical intervention can be considered. In 1947, Girdlestone transferred the flexor digitorum longus and brevis tendons into the dorsal expansions of the extensor tendons.[9] The theory was that the flexor muscles would take over the function of the lost intrinsic muscles. More commonly today, only the flexor digitorum longus tendon is transferred. There are multiple approaches for this tendon transfer depending on other procedures being concomitantly performed, the severity and complexity of the deformity, and surgeon preference. There are also other tendon transfers authors have described for digital and MTPJ deformities. This article will describe several techniques for the flexor digitorum longus tendon transfer and also review options for other tendon transfers for these complex problems.

As there is no gold standard for all digital deformities, it may be difficult to clearly define the absolute indication for the flexor digitorum longus tendon transfer. It may be utilized for a variety of situations and in combination with additional procedures. It is best considered as a useful adjunct if sequential hammertoe correction has failed to fully reduce the dorsal positioning of the proximal phalanx on the metatarsal head.

A flexor digitorum tendon transfer is indicated in patients with a floating digit and metatarsalgia. They may also have a dorsally contracted MTPJ, which can be manually reduced. As it has already been discussed that digital and MTPJ deformities can vary greatly, it can be deduced then that the surgical procedures available for their correction will also vary greatly. Lesser MTPJ instability is a challenging entity to correct in a lasting way. The myriad of biomechanical forces that cause it make it difficult to predict what combination of procedures will resolve the deformity most effectively. Typically, a combination of both osseous and soft tissue procedures is needed to gain sufficient surgical correction. Although there is great divergence in the strategies employed to treat digital and MTPJ deformities, the goal of the procedures is to reestablish alignment of the joint and digit.

It is not common to perform the flexor digitorum longus tendon transfer as a stand-alone procedure. Typically, the author will perform a proximal interphalangeal joint arthrodesis for digital stability. The plantar plate also needs to be assessed for rupture or attenuation. If either of these is found, then the plantar plate is also repaired. For long metatarsals, or if the surgeon cannot manually relocate the proximal phalanx adequately, the surgeon may need to perform a metatarsal osteotomy. This can be just a shortening and/or dorsiflexory osteotomy, or even a transpositional osteotomy for transverse plane correction. For a transverse plane deformity, soft tissue rebalancing of the collateral ligaments at the MTPJ may also be needed. For increased sagittal plane stability and alignment, the flexor digitorum longus tendon transfer is a good procedure.

Regardless of the approach for surgical reconstruction, for a lasting correction to be achieved, it must not only correct the existing anatomic deficiency, but also in some fashion alter the biomechanical tendency that caused the plantar plate to rupture in the first place. Care must be taken preoperatively when evaluating patients with lesser MTPJ instability for predisposing factors, because symptoms can persist postoperatively, despite correction of apparent deformity or the primary problem. Addressing these factors may help achieve a more predictable result by protecting the involved MTPJ from further deforming forces.

SURGICAL TECHNIQUE
Patient Preparation and Positioning

If the only surgical procedures to be performed are within the digital and MTPJ region, then the patient is usually placed in the supine position. The foot of the bed can be elevated in a Trendelenburg position if the surgeon needs access to the plantar aspect of the foot. The author typically uses an ankle tourniquet during the procedure to increase visualization. Anesthesia is usually intravenous sedation with local infiltrative blocks. If additional procedures, besides the forefoot, will be performed, the surgeon may opt for general or spinal anesthesia for more extensive or longer procedures.

FLEXOR DIGITORUM LONGUS TENDON TRANSFER (ONE INCISION)

When performing a concomitant hammertoe repair with the flexor tendon transfer, the flexor digitorum longus tendon is easily identified through the dorsal incision of the toe at the level of the proximal interphalangeal joint. A central dorsolinear incision is made from the metatarsal neck and ending at the middle phalanx. The incision can be curved over the MTPJ (**Fig. 4**A). The subcutaneous tissues are reflected, avoiding the neurovascular bundles medially and laterally. The extensor expansion is incised medially and laterally, and either a transverse tenotomy or lengthening of the extensor tendon is performed. Next, a sequential release of the MTPJ is performed. Plantar adhesions may also need to be released at this level with a McGlamry metatarsal elevator. Attention is then directed back to the proximal interphalangeal joint where the medial and lateral collateral ligaments are incised to expose the joint. If a proximal interphalangeal joint arthrodesis or arthroplasty is performed, the joint is prepared as per surgeon preference.

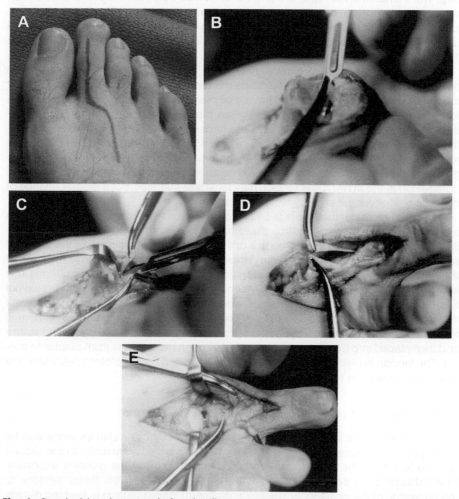

Fig. 4. One incisional approach for the flexor digitorum longus tendon transfer. Dorsal curvilinear incision (*A*). The flexor digitorum longus tendon is transected at the proximal interphalangeal joint. At this level, it is centrally located between the medial and lateral tendon slips of the flexor digitorum brevis (*B*). The flexor digitorum longus tendon is then split longitudinally into medial and lateral halves (*C*). The tendon halves are then brought proximally and dorsally around the proximal phalanx (*D*) and then sutured upon itself under physiologic tension (*E*).

The plantar tissue of the proximal interphalangeal joint is incised at the base of the middle phalanx. The flexor digitorum brevis tendon will be split into lateral and medial halves as they insert into the base of the middle phalanx. At this level, the flexor digitorum longus tendon will be located centrally between these tendon slips. The flexor digitorum longus tendon is then identified and isolated and transected within the proximal interphalangeal joint (**Fig. 4**B). The ankle can be plantarflexed to relieve tension on the flexor tendons. There are several techniques described to transfer the tendon. The standard technique, and the one the author routinely uses, is to split the flexor digitorum longus tendon into equal medial and lateral halves (**Fig. 4**C). Each of the tendon halves is then transferred proximally and dorsally around the proximal phalanx (**Fig. 4**D). If a hammertoe repair is being performed as well, then the proximal interphalangeal joint is fixated, utilizing the surgeons preferred method. The flexor digitorum longus tendon halves are then brought dorsally over the proximal phalanx and sutured together, typically with 3–0 non-absorbable suture, under physiologic tension (**Fig. 4**E).

The term physiologic tension in this scenario is really the surgeon's judgment of the proper amount of tension to be placed on the tendon to gain adequate correction of the digital and MTPJ deformities. The author deems appropriate tension is when the toe is still able to purchase the ground when the foot is weight bearing. Intraoperatively, the surgeon can place a flat surface under the foot and theoretically load the forefoot and simulate weight bearing. The digit should purchase this flat plate. If it is elevated, the tendon is probably under too much tension. More tension will give greater deformity correction, but there will be an increased risk of stiffness and limited dorsiflexion at the MTPJ. Less tension may have less stiffness, but a greater chance of deformity recurrence if stability is not achieved.

An alternate transfer method is to pass the full tendon from plantar to dorsal through a drill hole in the proximal phalanx. Kuwada and Dockery[10] described the flexor digitorum longus tendon transfer through a drill hole in the anatomic neck of the proximal phalanx, while Schuberth and Jensen[11] described it through a drill hole at the base of the proximal phalanx, stating it was a more anatomic approach. When utilizing this approach, the flexor digitorum longus tendon is transected at the level of the proximal interphalangeal joint, and a drill hole is placed in the base of the proximal phalanx directed from dorsal proximal to plantar distal. A wire loop is then placed in the drill hole from dorsal to plantar. The flexor digitorum longus tendon is tagged with suture and then placed into the wire loop and pulled through the drill hole from plantar to dorsal. The tendon is placed under physiologic tension and then a biotenodesis screw is utilized to secure the tendon in place.

FLEXOR DIGITORUM LONGUS TENDON TRANSFER (2 INCISIONS)

When this procedure is performed as an isolated procedure, 2 skin incisions can be employed. One incision is made on the side of the toe, typically medially on the second toe and lateral on the third, fourth, and fifth toes, to provide the greatest exposure. Sharp dissection is performed to open the retinacula binding the flexor tendons to the underside of the phalanges. The flexor digitorum longus tendon is severed distally near its attachment at the base of the distal phalanx. The longus tendon is then split longitudinally to the base of the proximal phalanx. A second incision is made dorsally and opposite the side of the initial incision on the proximal phalanx. A channel is created medially and laterally around the bone with a periosteal elevator, and then the tendon slips are drawn dorsally around the proximal phalanx and sutured upon themselves with 3–0 nonabsorbable suture.

FLEXOR DIGITORUM LONGUS TENDON TRANSFER (3 INCISIONS)

A 3-incision approach has also been described when there is no concomitant hammertoe deformity to be repaired. A small transverse incision is made plantarly at the crease of the MTPJ (**Fig. 5**A). The flexor digitorum longus tendon is identified and is the most plantar tendon at this level. A second transverse incision is made at

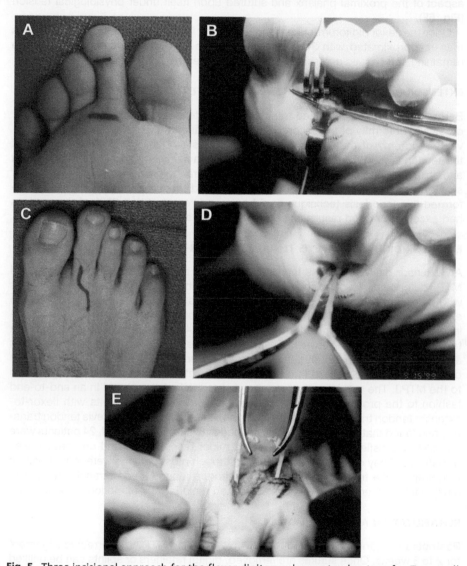

Fig. 5. Three incisional approach for the flexor digitorum longus tendon transfer. Two small transverse, plantar incisions at the crease of the distal interphalangeal joint and at the metatarsophalangeal joint (*A*). The flexor digitorum longus tendon is transected distally and then brought through the proximal plantar incision (*B*). A small curvilinear dorsal incision is made over the MTPJ (*C*). The flexor digitorum longus tendon is then split longitudinally in the plantar incision (*D*), and then the medial and lateral tendon halves are brought through the dorsal incision and sutured upon itself on the dorsum of the proximal phalanx (*E*).

the plantar crease of the distal interphalangeal joint. The flexor digitorum longus tendon is transected at its insertion into the base of the distal phalanx and then brought proximally into the proximal incision (**Fig. 5**B). A small curvilinear incision is then made on the dorsum of the foot over the MTPJ, and a dorsal MTPJ capsulotomy is performed (**Fig. 5**C). The flexor digitorum longus tendon is split in half longitudinally (**Fig. 5**D), and the tendon halves are transferred medially and laterally to the dorsal aspect of the proximal phalanx and sutured upon itself under physiological tension (**Fig. 5**E).

Once the flexor digitorum longus tendon transfer is complete, the extensor tendon is then reapproximated with 3–0 absorbable suture, and then layered closure of the remaining soft tissues and skin is performed as per the surgeon's preference.

EXTENSOR DIGITORUM LONGUS TENDON TRANSFER

Barca and Acciaro[12] described transfer of the extensor digitorum longus tendon for crossover deformity of the second toe. They release the MTPJ and perform a transverse tenotomy of the extensor digitorum longus tendon. The proximal portion of the tendon is then threaded under the intermetatarsal ligament between the second and third metatarsal heads and placed into a drill hole on the lateral and plantar side of the base of the proximal phalanx directed medially and dorsally. They performed this tenodesis technique on 30 toes and reported that 83% of the patients had excellent or good results (excellent in 10 toes and good in 15 toes).

EXTENSOR DIGITORUM BREVIS TENDON TRANSFER

An extensor digitorum brevis tendon transfer can also be performed for digital and MTPJ deformities. Haddad and colleagues[13] performed this procedure on 19 patients with crossover second toe deformity. The MTPJ is dissected and released, and the extensor digitorum brevis tendon is dissected proximally. Two stay sutures are inserted into the extensor digitorum brevis tendon 4 cm proximal to the MTPJ, and a tenotomy is performed between these sutures. The distal end of the tendon remains attached to the extensor hood apparatus, and then the distal stump is routed, from distal to proximal, plantar to the deep transverse intermetatarsal ligament and lateral to the MTPJ. The extensor digitorum brevis tendon is then sutured in an end-to-end fashion to the proximal portion. This analysis compared 16 patients with flexor-to-extensor tendon transfers and 19 patients with extensor digitorum brevis tendon transfers and found that both treatment groups had similar results. Overall, 24 patients were completely satisfied; 6 patients had some minor reservations, and one patient was dissatisfied. They did state however, that although most patients were free of pain at follow-up, those treated with the flexor digitorum longus tendon transfer tended to have more pain, and those with more pain had residual lack of motion at the MTPJ.

REHABILITATION AND RECOVERY

Postoperative bandaging is used to retain the toes and MTPJs in corrected alignment for 2 to 3 weeks. Once sutures are removed, digital retainers or splints can be utilized to maintain alignment. This is typically utilized for an additional 4 to 8 weeks while osseous healing continues. Patients are usually partial weight bearing on their heel in a surgical shoe during the healing time. Once pain and swelling permit, they can progress to a regular shoe and return to normal activities. Range-of-motion exercises of the MTPJ can also be employed about 2 to 3 weeks postoperatively to try to minimize stiffness of the joint.

COMPLICATIONS

The greatest patient complaint regarding the flexor digitorum longus tendon transfer is stiffness. Some stiffness, however, will help reduce the risk of recurrence of deformity. The surgeon has to know the proper amount of physiologic tension to utilize during the transfer to help minimize the recurrence rate yet maintain necessary motion. On the other hand, one could also get overcorrection and get a reverse deformity if too much tension is applied during the transfer. Other complications include loss of active flexion and fracture of the proximal phalanx if using a drill hole for the tendon transfer. Classic complications associated with traditional hammertoe repair, such as angular deformities, floating toe, lack of toe purchase, prolonged edema, scarring, numbness, and vascular insult, can also occur.

CLINICAL RESULTS IN THE LITERATURE

The literature is controversial regarding the flexor digitorum longus tendon transfer. Some surgeons avoid the procedure, stating that the toe becomes too stiff after the surgery; others, however, state that part of the success in the procedure is the stiffness it produces, because there is less chance of recurrence.

Transfer of the flexor digitorum longus tendon for correction of digital deformities was described by Trethowan[14] in 1925. Girdlestone[9] used the procedure years before Taylor described it in 1951 as the transfer of the long and short flexor tendons to the extensor expansion, and it became known as the Girdlestone-Taylor procedure.[15] Parrish then modified the procedure to include splitting the flexor tendon longitudinally and suturing the ends to themselves and to the dorsal extensor tendon expansion[16] Taylor reported performing the Girdelstone procedure on 112 feet.[15] He followed 68 of the cases and reported 59 good results. Pyper[17] reviewed 45 feet that underwent a flexor tendon transfer and reported an equal number of good and poor results. He had a higher success in milder deformities and recommended a proximal interphalangeal joint arthrodesis as a better alternative.

Sgarlato[18] reported on 53 cases of flexor tendon transfers utilizing 2 different techniques and reported that one toe was elevated and edematous. Barbari and Brevig[19] reported on 39 operations in 31 patients. They noted satisfactory results in 28 patients. They also stated that when metatarsalgia was the primary preoperative complaint, no improvement was noted postoperatively.

Mendicino and colleagues[20] performed a retrospective analysis on 8 patients who received a flexor tendon transfer and had excellent results in 6 patients. Residual stiffness was the primary complaint of 2 patients following the procedure. Myerson and Jung[21] treated 64 feet with a split flexor digitorum longus tendon transfer and performed a retrospective analysis. Results included 26 patients who were satisfied, 15 patients who were satisfied with minor reservations, 6 patients who were satisfied with major reservations, and 12 patients who were not satisfied. Additional procedures, including MTPJ capsulotomy, collateral ligament release, extensor tendon lengthening, metatarsal osteotomy, and hammertoe repair were performed as the surgeon deemed appropriate. They concluded that many patients were not satisfied, mostly because of residual stiffness, loss of active flexion, and dysfunction. It should be noted that the authors did not address the plantar plate in this study, and only 9 feet had a proximal interphalangeal joint arthrodesis. The author believes these could be reasons for the patient dissatisfaction.

Boyer and DeOrio[22] reported an 89% satisfaction rate, 70 out of 79 toes, for the flexor-to-extensor tendon transfer. They reported no floating toes, high patient satisfaction, and few complications with the procedure. Bouche and Heit[23] retrospectively evaluated a case series of 18 patients with the combined procedures of plantar plate repair, hammertoe repair, and flexor digitorum longus tendon transfer. All patients were satisfied with their postoperative result, and they concluded that this combination of procedures was a viable option to address severe, chronic sagittal plane instability of the lesser MTPJs. Postoperative complaints included digital stiffness in 40% of patients (6 patients), mild joint pain in 33% of patients (5 patients), localized digital numbness in 13% of patients (2 patients), and swelling in 13% of patients (2 patients). They also stated that it is important to reestablish both static and dynamic stabilization of the digit. The plantar plate repair provides static stabilization, and the flexor digitorum longus tendon transfer should provide dynamic stability.

Iglesias and colleagues[24] performed a meta-analysis of the flexor tendon transfer with the aim of the study to evaluate the clinical benefit of the procedure. Two hundred three articles were retrieved, and 17 publications met the inclusion and exclusion criteria and were entered into the analysis. Overall patient satisfaction with the procedure was 86.7%. When adjusting for higher-quality prospective studies, overall patient satisfaction was increased to 91.8%. They concluded that there was supportive evidence of the clinical benefit of the flexor digitorum longus tendon transfer. They also found that there was no significant difference of success of the procedure regarding the age and sex of the patient. They further found that the most common reason for an unsatisfied patient was stiffness, and better satisfaction rates were found in toes that also had a proximal interphalangeal joint arthrodesis performed in addition to the tendon transfer.

Ford and colleagues[25] performed a cadaveric study comparing plantar plate repair with flexor digitorum longus tendon transfer. Although they felt that the flexor digitorum longus tendon transfer was a good procedure, they reasoned that a combined flexor digitorum longus tendon transfer and plantar plate repair for subluxed and dislocated joints would be most effective for stabilizing the MTPJ.

Chalayon and colleagues[26] also performed a cadaver-based study and concluded that when the plantar plate was disrupted, there was significant instability in the lesser MTPJ. They concluded that the flexor-to-extensor tendon transfer by itself increased stability of the joint in dorsiflexion, but when combined with the Weil osteotomy it restored near-intact stability against superior subluxation and dorsiflexion forces.

The flexor digitorum brevis tendon has also been described to aid in stabilizing the MTPJ. Maestro and colleagues[27] described the Pisani technique and stated that it was more difficult than the flexor digitorum longus tendon transfer because of the smaller diameter of the tendon but is more logical, because the flexor digitorum longus tendon transfer leads to residual stiffness.

SUMMARY

Complex digital deformities and metatarsophalangeal joint instability encompass a wide range of pathology. Digital and metatarsophalangeal joint deformities are common and unfortunately can be challenging for the foot and ankle surgeon. The surgical treatment for these complex deformities should be individualized and requires a sequential process for adequate reduction and deformity correction. The flexor digitorum longus tendon transfer is just one option and typically just one part of a multitude of procedures that may include proximal interphalangeal joint arthrodesis, soft tissue rebalancing, plantar plate repair, other tendon transfers, and a metatarsal osteotomy. Because of the complexity of the deformity and the multiplanes that can be involved, there is no one procedure that is the gold standard for every deformity. The flexor digitorum longus tendon transfer is a common and popular procedure to help aid in reestablishing mechanical stability to the MTPJ. It changes the deforming force of the flexor digitorum longus to one of active stabilization and plantarflexion of the proximal phalanx at the MTPJ. Although residual stiffness can result from the flexor digitorum longus tendon transfer, overall patient satisfaction levels remain high when it is performed under the proper indications and concomitantly with other procedures to gain full correction of these challenging deformities.

There is a video that accompanies this article. It shows the technique utilized and described by the author for the one incisional approach for the flexor digitorum longus tendon transfer. The video was produced by Trent K. Statler, DPM, FACFAS (Video 1).

SUPPLEMENTARY DATA

Supplementary data related to this article can be found online at http://dx.doi.org/10.1016/j.cpm.2015.06.015.

REFERENCES

1. Yu GV, Judge MS. Predislocation syndrome of the lesser metatarsophalangeal joint: a distinct clinical entity. In: Camasta CA, Vickers NS, Carter SR, editors. Reconstructive surgery of the foot and leg update '95. Tucker (GA): The Podiatry Institute; 1995. p. 109.
2. Yu GV, Judge MS, Hudson JR, et al. Predislocation syndrome: progressive subluxation/dislocation of the lesser metatarsophalangeal joint. J Am Podiatr Med Assoc 2002;92:182–99.
3. Bhatia D, Myerson MS, Curtis MJ, et al. Anatomical restraints to dislocation of the second metatarsophalangeal joint and assessment of repair technique. J Bone Joint Surg Am 1994;76:1371.
4. Gregg J, Silberstein M, Schneider T, et al. Sonographic and MRI evaluation of the plantar plate: a prospective study. Eur Radiol 2006;16:2661–9.
5. Fortin PT, Myerson MS. Second metatarsophalangeal joint instability. Foot Ankle Int 1995;16:306–13.
6. Trepman F, Yeo S. Nonoperative treatment of the second metatarsophalangeal joint synovitis. Foot Ankle Int 1995;16:771–7.
7. Mizel MS, Michelson JD. Nonsurgical treatment of monoarticular nontraumatic synovitis of the second metatarsophalangeal joint. Foot Ankle Int 1997;18:424–6.
8. Reis ND, Karkabi S, Zinman C. Metatarsophalangeal joint dislocation after local steroid injection. J Bone Joint Surg Br 1989;71:864.
9. Girdlestone GR. Physiotherapy for hand and foot. Physiotherapy 1947;32:167.
10. Kuwada GT, Dockery GL. Modification of the flexor tendon transfer procedure for the correction of flexible hammertoes. J Foot Surg 1980;19:38.
11. Schuberth JM, Jensen R. Flexor digitorum longus transfer for second metatarsophalangeal joint dislocation/subluxation. In: Vickers NS, Miller SJ, Mahan KT, et al, editors. Reconstructive surgery of the foot and leg update '97. Tucker (GA): The Podiatry Institute; 1997. p. 11–4.
12. Barca F, Acciaro AL. Surgical correction of crossover deformity of the second toe: a technique for tenodesis. Foot Ankle Int 2003;42(4):178–82.
13. Haddad SL, Sabbagh RC, Resch S, et al. Results of flexor-to extensor and extensor brevis tendon transfer for correction of the crossover second toe deformity. Foot Ankle Int 1999;20(12):781–8.
14. Trethowan WH. The treatment of hammertoe. Lancet 1925;1:1312.
15. Taylor RG. The treatment of claw toes by multiple transfers of flexor into extensor tendons. J Bone Joint Surg Br 1951;33:539.

16. Parrish TF. Dynamic correction of clawtoes. Orthop Clin North Am 1973;4:97.
17. Pyper JB. The flexor-extensor transplant operation for claw toes. J Bone Joint Surg Br 1958;40:528–33.
18. Sgarlato TE. Transplantation of the flexor digitorum longus muscle tendon in hammertoes. J Am Podiatry Assoc 1970;60:383–8.
19. Barbari SG, Brevig K. Correction of clawtoes by the Girdlestone–Taylor flexor–extensor transfer procedure. Foot Ankle 1984;5:67–73.
20. Mendicino RW, Statler TK, Saltrick KR, et al. Predislocation syndrome: a review and retrospective analysis of eight patients. J Foot Ankle Surg 2001;40:214–24.
21. Myerson MS, Jung HG. The role of toe flexor-to-extensor transfer in correcting metatarsophalangeal joint instability of the second toe. Foot Ankle Int 2005;26:675–9.
22. Boyer ML, DeOrio JK. Transfer of the flexor digitorum longus for the correction of lesser toe deformities. Foot Ankle Int 2007;28:422–30.
23. Bouche RT, Heit EJ. Combined plantar plate and hammertoe repair with flexor digitorum longus tendon transfer for chronic, severe sagittal plane instability of the lesser metatarsophalangeal joints: preliminary observations. J Foot Ankle Surg 2008;47:125–37.
24. Iglesias ME, Vallejo RB, Jules KT, et al. Meta-analysis of flexor tendon transfer for the correction of lesser toe deformities. J Am Podiatr Med Assoc 2012;102:359–68.
25. Ford LA, Collins KB, Christensen JC. Stabilization of the subluxed second metatarsophalangeal joint: flexor tendon transfer versus primary repair of the plantar plate. J Foot Ankle Surg 1998;37:375–8.
26. Chalayon O, Chertman C, Guss AD, et al. Role of plantar plate and surgical reconstruction techniques on static stability of lesser metatarsophalangeal joints: a biomechanical study. Foot Ankle Int 2013;34:1346–442.
27. Maestro M, Ferre B, Cazal J. Flexor digitorum brevis (FDB) transfer (Pisani technique) in correcting metatarsophalangeal joint (MPJ) instability of the second toe. J Orthop Trauma Surg and Related Research 2010;18:50–2.

Tendon Transfers and Salvaging Options for Hallux Varus Deformities

Brian P. Gradisek, DPM*, Lowell Weil Jr, DPM, MBA

KEYWORDS

- Hallux varus • Tendon transfer • Varus deformity • Varus repair

KEY POINTS

- Hallux varus deformity is most commonly seen as an iatrogenic complication of hallux valgus surgery.
- Tendon transfers are a viable option for correction of flexible hallux varus deformity.
- There have been many soft tissue–balancing procedures described for treatment of flexible hallux varus; however, it remains unclear which procedure is the most advantageous and sustainable.

INTRODUCTION

Hallux varus is an infrequently encountered deformity of the first ray characterized by a medial deviation of the hallux on the first metatarsal head at the first metatarsal phalangeal joint (MPJ), as seen in **Figs. 1** and **2**.[1] Although this condition may be congenital, it is most commonly seen as an iatrogenic complication of bunion surgery resulting from an overcorrection of hallux valgus.[2,3]

Causes of iatrogenic hallux varus include overtightening of the medial capsule combined with an excessive lateral release leading to an imbalance of the soft tissues and unopposed pull of the medial musculature on the hallux. In addition, there may be loss of osseous support at the medial aspect of the MPJ because of excessive bone resection or overcorrection of the intermetatarsal angle. Excision of the fibular sesamoid may allow the hallux to drift into a varus position.[1,2,4] Finally, overcorrection of hallux interphalangeus with a medial closing wedge phalangeal osteotomy (Akin) may cause a medially directed pull of the extensor hallucis longus (EHL) and flexor hallucis longus (FHL) pulling the hallux into a varus position.[5]

The authors have nothing to disclose related to the content of this chapter.
Weil Foot & Ankle Institute, Des Plaines, IL, USA
* Corresponding author. 1400 28th Street, Suite 2, Boulder, CO 80303.
E-mail address: bgradisek@gmail.com

Clin Podiatr Med Surg 33 (2016) 85–98
http://dx.doi.org/10.1016/j.cpm.2015.06.008
0891-8422/16/$ – see front matter © 2016 Elsevier Inc. All rights reserved.
podiatric.theclinics.com

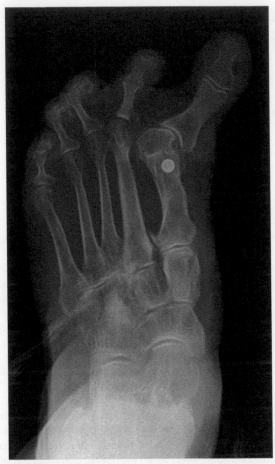

Fig. 1. Anteroposterior (AP) radiograph demonstrating iatrogenic hallux varus deformity.

Iatrogenic flexible hallux varus often requires surgical repair to create a functional, pain-free, shoeable foot. There have been many procedures described to facilitate this repair; however, it remains unclear which procedure is the most advantageous and sustainable. Fusion of the first MPJ (**Fig. 3**) has been shown to be the most durable procedure to correct hallux valgus, but joint functionality is compromised.[5,6] This article describes the soft tissue procedures that may be used to correct flexible hallux varus deformity while preserving the function of the first MPJ.

INDICATION

A tendon transfer procedure as treatment of hallux varus is reserved for cases of flexible deformity with a functioning and painless first MPJ. Correcting the deformity through the use of a joint-sparing soft tissue procedure may prevent occurrence of degenerative arthrosis and motion loss of the MPJ.[7] Cases of hallux varus deformity with concurrent degeneration of the first MPJ will not respond well to soft tissue transfer procedures, and arthrodesis should be considered.[8] The joint should be evaluated radiographically and clinically before surgical decision-making.

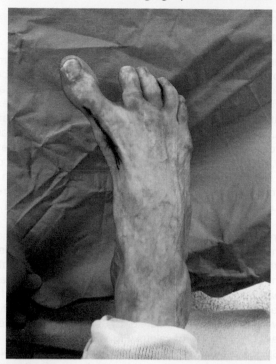

Fig. 2. Hallux varus deformity.

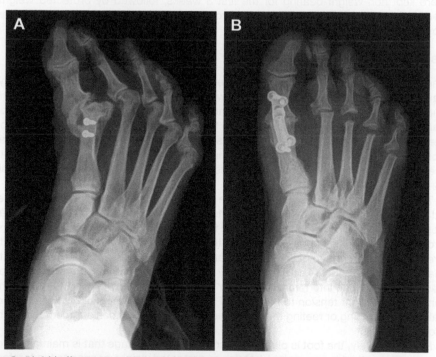

Fig. 3. Rigid hallux varus with joint destruction treated with fusion of the first MPJ. (*A*) AP radiograph demonstrating iatrogenic hallux varus with joint destruction. (*B*) AP radiograph of same patient after first MPJ fusion with plate and screws.

EXTENSOR HALLUCIS LONGUS TRANSFER

The EHL tendon transfer for repair of flexible hallux valgus is a dynamic transfer orig-inally described by Johnson and Spiegl[9] in 1984. The patient is placed in the supine position and standard preparation and drape are performed. A dorsal L-shaped inci-sion is made beginning between the first and second metatarsals, extending distally along the dorsolateral aspect of the great toe and angled medially at the insertion of the EHL. The EHL is then resected off the base of the proximal phalanx as far distally as possible with care taken to avoid disruption of the nail bed. The end of the EHL tendon is tagged, and the paratenon is freed proximally. A medial capsular release is necessary and may be performed through the joint or through an ancillary medial incision. The articular surfaces of the first interphalangeal joint are then resected and an intermedullary bone screw is driven from distal to proximal to fuse the joint in extension.

The EHL tendon is then passed from proximal to distal, plantar to the intermetatarsal ligament between the heads of the first and second metatarsals. This technique uses the intermetatarsal ligament as a pulley to redirect the force applied by the EHL tendon. A 3.5-mm drill is used to create a tunnel from dorsal to plantar in the base of the first proximal phalanx. The tendon is then passed from plantar to dorsal through the tunnel. The tendon may be secured under slight tension by suturing the tendon back on to itself with nonabsorbable suture or by using an interference or biotenodesis screw with the hallux in 5° to 15° of valgus (**Fig. 4**).

Johnson and Spiegl[9] advocated crossed Kirschner wires to be placed across the first MPJ to hold correction along with cast immobilization for 6 weeks. The patients were kept non-weight-bearing for the first 3 weeks, followed by protected weight-bearing for 3 weeks. K-wire removal, unprotected weight-bearing, and physical ther-apy occur at 6 weeks.

ABDUCTOR HALLUCIS TRANSFER

The abductor hallucis (ABH) tendon transfer for repair of flexible hallux valgus is a dy-namic transfer originally described by Hawkins[3] in 1971. The patient is placed in the supine position and standard preparation and drape are performed. A linear longitudi-nal dorsomedial incision is made over the first MPJ. The ABH tendon is resected off the medial sesamoid and the medial base of the proximal phalanx as distally as possible to maintain maximum length of the tendon. A whipstitch is performed about the end of the tendon, and the paratenon is freed proximally. A medial release is per-formed at the MPJ.

The tendon is then passed plantar to the first metatarsal neck into the first interme-tatarsal space and then distally plantar to the intermetatarsal ligament. Using an appropriately sized drill, a tunnel is created from lateral to medial in the base of the first proximal phalanx. It is important to center this tunnel on the neutral line of the bone to prevent pronation or supination of the phalanx. The tendon is passed from lateral to medial into the tunnel. There is typically insufficient length to suture the tendon back on itself, so an interference screw or biotenodesis screw is used to secure the tendon under slight tension to the base of the phalanx with the hallux in 5° to 15° of valgus. Reattaching or reefing the conjoined adductor tendon can augment this tech-nique (**Fig. 5**).

Postoperatively, the foot is placed in a compressive bandage that is maintained for 1 week. The patient is non-weight-bearing or protected weight-bearing to the forefoot for 6 weeks. Physical therapy begins at 1 week postoperatively to maintain range of motion and strengthen the musculature. Syndactylization to the second toe with

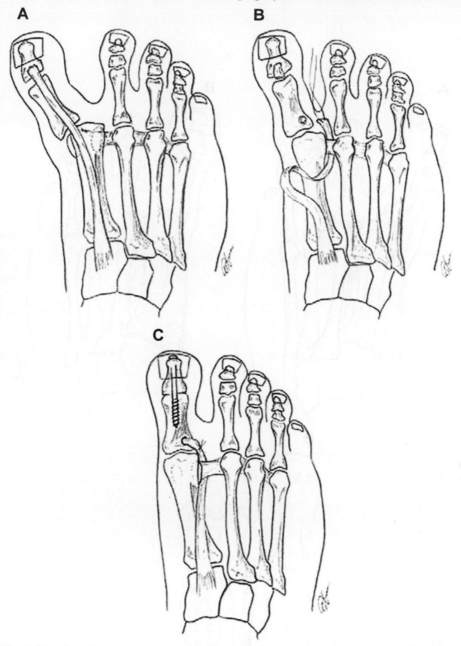

Fig. 4. Transfer of the EHL tendon to the base of the proximal phalanx of the hallux with interphalangeal arthrodesis. (*A*) Preoperative depiction of the position of the FHL tendon in the presence of hallux varus deformity. (*B*) After a medial soft tissue release, the MPJ becomes reducible. The EHL tendon is released from its insertion at the distal phalanx of the hallux. The tendon is tagged and passed inferior to the intermetatarsal ligament. A dorsal-to-plantar tunnel is drilled in the base of the proximal phalanx of the hallux. (*C*) The EHL tendon is passed through the osseous tunnel from plantar to dorsal and sutured on itself under slight tension. An interphalangeal arthrodesis of the hallux is performed as necessary. (*Courtesy of* C. Husson; and *From* Bevernage BD, Leemrijse T. Hallux varus: classification and treatment. Foot Ankle Clin 2009;14:59; with permission.)

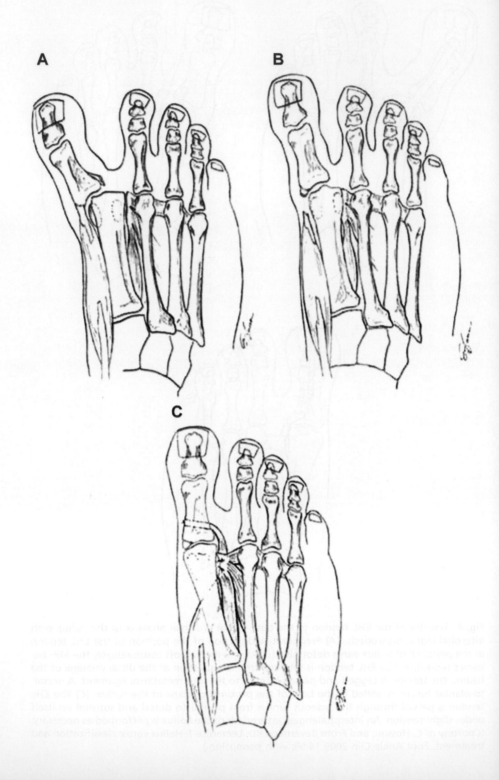

self-adherent elastic wrap is maintained for 8 weeks to maintain position while healing occurs.[5,10]

FIRST DORSAL INTEROSSEOUS TRANSFER

The first dorsal interosseous tendon transfer for repair of flexible hallux valgus is a dynamic transfer originally described by Valtin[11] in 1991. The patient is placed in the supine position and standard preparation and drape are performed. A linear longitudinal dorsomedial or dorsolateral incision is made over the first MPJ. A medial capsular and abductor release or lengthening is performed. The first dorsal interosseous muscle and tendon are identified within the first intermetatarsal space. The tendon is resected at the insertion into the base of the second proximal phalanx. A whipstitch is performed about the distal end of the tendon.

A tunnel is created from lateral to medial in the base of the proximal phalanx with an appropriately sized drill. It is important to center this tunnel on the neutral line of the bone to prevent pronation or supination of the phalanx. The tendon is then passed dorsal to the intermetatarsal ligament and into the tunnel created in the proximal phalanx. The tendon may be secured under slight tension by suturing the tendon back onto itself or by using an interference or biotenodesis screw with the hallux in 5° to 15° of valgus (**Fig. 6**). Reattaching or reefing the conjoined adductor tendon can augment this technique.

Postoperatively, the foot is placed in a compressive bandage that is maintained for 1 week. The patient is non-weight-bearing or protected weight-bearing to the forefoot for 6 weeks. Physical therapy begins at 1 week postoperatively to maintain range of motion and strengthen the musculature. Syndactylization to the second toe with self-adherent elastic wrap is maintained for 8 weeks to maintain position while healing occurs.[5,10]

SPLIT EXTENSOR HALLUCIS LONGUS TRANSFER

The split EHL tendon transfer for repair of flexible hallux valgus is a static transfer originally described by Lau and Myerson in 2002.[11,12] The patient is placed in the supine position and standard preparation and drape are performed. A linear longitudinal dorsomedial incision is made over the first MPJ. A medial capsular and abductor release or lengthening is performed. The lateral half of the EHL tendon is detached proximally near the base of the first metatarsal. A whipstitch is performed about the proximal end of the lateral half of the EHL tendon. The detached lateral half of the tendon is then passed from distal to proximal under intermetatarsal ligament in the first intermetatarsal space.

Fig. 5. Transfer of the ABH tendon to the base of the proximal phalanx of the hallux with reattachment of the adductor hallucis tendon to the lateral sesamoid. (*A*) Preoperative depiction of the position of the ABH tendon in the presence of hallux varus deformity and medial adductor tendon release. (*B*) A medial release is performed and the ABH tendon is released at its insertion to the medial base of the proximal phalanx as distally as possible to maintain maximum length of the tendon. The adductor tendon is reattached to the lateral sesamoid. (*C*) The abductor tendon is passed inferior to the adductor tendon and intermetatarsal ligament and passed from lateral to medial through the osseous tunnel and secured under slight tension. (*Courtesy of* C. Husson; and *From* Bevernage BD, Leemrijse T. Hallux varus: classification and treatment. Foot Ankle Clin 2009;14:58; with permission.)

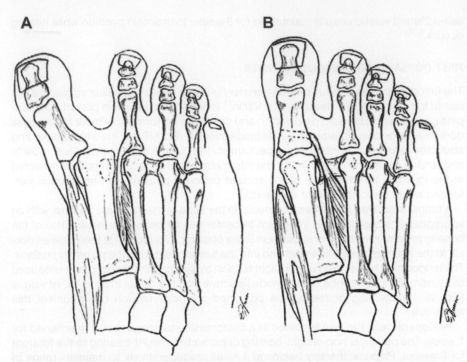

Fig. 6. Transfer of the first dorsal interosseous tendon to the base of the proximal phalanx of the hallux. (*A*) Preoperative depiction of the position of the ABH tendon and first dorsal interosseous tendon in the presence of hallux varus deformity. (*B*) After a medial release, the first dorsal interosseous tendon is released from its insertion to the base of the second proximal phalanx. The tendon is transferred into an osseous tunnel from lateral to medial in the base of the proximal phalanx of the hallux under slight tension. (*Courtesy of* C. Husson; and *From* Bevernage BD, Leemrijse T. Hallux varus: classification and treatment. Foot Ankle Clin 2009;14:59; with permission.)

A tunnel is created in the neck of the first metatarsal from medial to lateral with an appropriately sized drill. The lateral half of the EHL tendon is then passed from lateral to medial through the tunnel in the first metatarsal. The tendon may be secured under slight tension by suturing the tendon back on to itself or by using an interference or tenodesis screw with the hallux in 5° to –15° of valgus. This repair will have a supinating effect while laterally deviating the hallux (**Fig. 7**).

Postoperatively, the foot is placed in a compressive bandage that is maintained for 1 week. The patient is non-weight-bearing or protected weight-bearing to the forefoot for 6 weeks. Physical therapy begins at 1 week postoperatively to maintain range of motion and strengthen the musculature. Syndactylization to the second toe with self-adherent elastic wrap is maintained for 8 weeks to maintain position while healing occurs.[5,10]

REVERSE ABDUCTOR HALLUCIS TRANSFER

The reverse ABH tendon transfer for repair of flexible hallux valgus is a static transfer originally described by Leemrijse and colleagues[10] in 2008. The patient is placed in the supine position and standard preparation and drape are performed. A linear

A   B

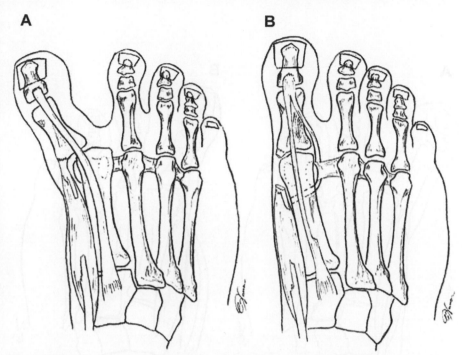

Fig. 7. Modified split EHL tendon transfer to the first metatarsal. (A) Preoperative depiction of the position of the EHL tendon in the presence of hallux varus deformity. (B) A medial release the EHL tendon is split, maintaining the insertion to the distal phalanx of the hallux. The lateral half of the EHL tendon is passed inferior to the intermetatarsal ligament and passed from lateral to medial through an osseous tunnel in the neck of the first metatarsal and sutured in place under slight tension. (*Courtesy of* C. Husson; and *From* Bevernage BD, Leemrijse T. Hallux varus: classification and treatment. Foot Ankle Clin 2009;14:62; with permission.)

longitudinal medial incision is made at the first MPJ, and a medial release is performed. The ABH tendon is resected proximally at the musculotendinous junction, keeping the distal attachment to the first proximal phalanx intact. The attachment of the ABH tendon to the medial sesamoid must also be released. A whipstitch is performed about the proximal end of the ABH tendon.

An oblique osseous tunnel is created with an appropriately sized drill in the base of the first proximal phalanx from distal medial to proximal lateral, beginning a few millimeters distal to the insertion of the ABH tendon. It is important to center this tunnel on the neutral line of the bone to prevent pronation or supination of the phalanx. A second oblique osseous tunnel is created in the neck of the first metatarsal from proximal medial to distal lateral. The tendon first is passed from medial to lateral through the tunnel in the proximal phalanx. An ancillary incision in the first web space is performed to facilitate the passage of the tendon. The tendon is recovered in the first web space passed superior to the intermetatarsal ligament, and through the tunnel in the first metatarsal from lateral to medial (**Fig. 8**).

The transferred tendon is then sutured to the periosteum and the remaining fibers of the ABH at the medial aspect of the first metatarsal using transosseous

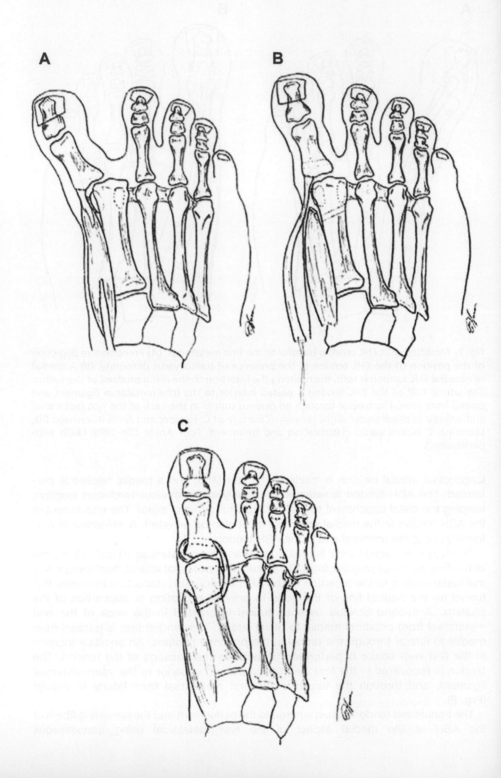

nonabsorbable suture. The tendon is secured with slight tension and 5° to 15° valgus position of the hallux.

Postoperatively, the foot is placed in a compressive bandage that is maintained for 1 week. The patient is non-weight-bearing or protected weight-bearing to the forefoot for 6 weeks. Physical therapy begins at 1 week postoperatively to maintain range of motion and strengthen the musculature. Syndactylization to the second toe with self-adherent elastic wrap is maintained for 8 weeks to maintain position while healing occurs.[5,10]

EXTENSOR HALLUCIS BREVIS TENODESIS

The extensor hallucis brevis (EHB) tenodesis for repair of flexible hallux valgus is a static transfer originally described by Myerson and Komenda in 1996.[13] The patient is placed in the supine position and standard preparation and drape are performed. A linear longitudinal dorsomedial incision is made at the first MPJ and a medial release is performed. The EHB tendon is identified distally and traced proximally to the myo-tendinous junction, where it is tagged with suture and transected, leaving the distal attachment intact.

An oblique osseous tunnel is created in the first metatarsal with an appropriately sized drill. The osseous tunnel begins 1.5 cm proximal to the MPJ and is directed from dorsomedial proximal to plantar lateral distal. The tendon is passed from distal to proximal, inferior to the intermetatarsal ligament, which will serve as a fulcrum to pull the hallux out of extension and out of its varus position (**Fig. 9**). The tendon is then passed through the osseous tunnel and secured under slight tension using an interference screw or biotenodesis screw with the hallux in 5° to 15° of valgus.[14]

Postoperatively, the foot is placed in a compressive bandage that is maintained for 1 week. The patient is non-weight-bearing or protected weight-bearing to the forefoot for 6 weeks. Physical therapy begins at 1 week postoperatively to maintain range of motion and strengthen the musculature. Syndactylization to the second toe with self-adherent elastic wrap is maintained for 8 weeks to maintain position while healing occurs.[5,10]

Fig. 8. Reversed ABH tendon transfer to the first metatarsal. (*A*) Preoperative depiction of the position of the ABH tendon in the presence of hallux varus deformity. (*B*) After a medial release, the ABH tendon is resected proximally at the musculotendinous junction, keeping the distal attachment to the first proximal phalanx intact. The proximal end of the ABH tendon is tagged with suture. An oblique osseous tunnel is created from distal medial to proximal lateral in the base of the first proximal phalanx. A second oblique osseous tunnel is created in the neck of the first metatarsal from proximal medial to distal lateral. (*C*) The ABH tendon is passed from medial to lateral through the osseous tunnel in the proximal phalanx and then from lateral to medial through the osseous tunnel in the first metatarsal and secured medially with suture. Note that the tendon is passed superior to the intermetatarsal ligament. (*Courtesy of* C. Husson; and *From* Bevernage BD, Leemrijse T. Hallux varus: classification and treatment. Foot Ankle Clin 2009;14:61; with permission.)

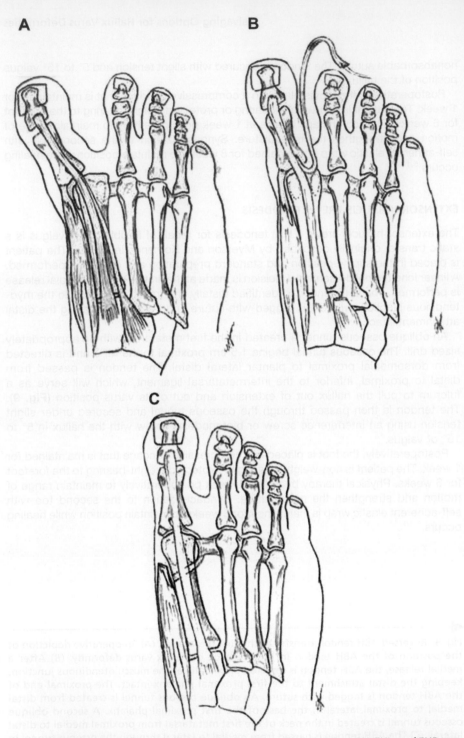

Fig. 9. EHB tenodesis. (*A*) Preoperative depiction of the position of the ABH, EHL, and EHB tendons in the presence of hallux varus deformity. (*B*) The EHB tendon is transected near the base of the first metatarsal and tagged with suture. (*C*) A medial release the EHB tendon is passed from distal to proximal, inferior to the intermetatarsal ligament, and secured into an osseous tunnel in the first metatarsal. (*Courtesy of* C. Husson; and *From* Bevernage BD, Leemrijse T. Hallux varus: classification and treatment. Foot Ankle Clin 2009;14:63; with permission.)

SUMMARY

Flexible hallux varus is an uncommon result of hallux valgus surgery that often requires surgical repair to create a painless congruent joint and a shoeable foot. Many soft tissue procedures have been described as treatment of hallux varus, and because most of the literature consists of retrospective case studies, the most advantageous soft tissue procedure remains unknown. Prospective head-to-head comparison of these procedures must be undertaken to identify the most viable and sustainable technique. New techniques using a synthetic suture button construct to re-create the lateral collateral ligament of the first MPJ have been recently described and seem to be a viable alternative to tendon transfer.[15]

Arthrodesis remains the mainstay of treatment because it is commonly thought that soft tissue procedures will ultimately fail. However, a systematic review of the literature by Plonavich and colleagues[16] recently found that soft tissue procedures seem to be an acceptable option with predictable results for the first-line treatment of iatrogenic flexible hallux varus. Arthrodesis should be reserved for cases of recalcitrant hallux varus with damage to the MPJ.

REFERENCES

1. Janis LR, Donick II. The etiology of hallux varus: a review. J Am Podiatr Med Assoc 1975;65:233–7.
2. Edelman RD. Iatrogenically induced hallux varus. Clin Podiatr Med Surg 1991;8: 367–82.
3. Hawkins FB. Acquired hallux valgus: cause, prevention and correction. Clin Orthop Relat Res 1971;76:169–76.
4. Zahari D, Girolamo M. Hallux varus: a step-wise approach for correction. J Foot Surg 1991;30:264–6.
5. Bevernage BD, Leemrijse T. Hallux varus: classification and treatment. Foot Ankle Clin 2009;14:51–65.
6. Goldman FD, Siegel J, Barton C. Extensor hallucis longus tendon transfer for correction of hallux varus. J Foot Ankle Surg 1993;32:126–31.
7. Maynou C, Beltrand E, Podglajen J, et al. Utilisation des Transferts Tendineux dans les Hallux Varus Post Op_eratoires. Rev Chir Orthop Reparatrice Appar Mot 2000;86:181–7.
8. Geaney LE, Myerson MS. Radiographic results after hallux metatarsophalangeal joint arthrodesis for hallux varus. Foot Ankle Int 2015;36(4): 391–4.
9. Johnson KA, Spiegl PV. Extensor hallucis longus transfer for hallux varus deformity. J Bone Joint Surg Am 1984;66(5):681–6.
10. Leemrijse Th, Hoang B, Maldague P, et al. A new surgical procedure for iatrogenic hallux varus: reverse transfer of the abductor hallucis tendon. A report of 7 cases. Acta Orthop Belg 2008;74:227–34.
11. Valtin B. Le transfert du premier Interosseus dorsal dans le Traitoment Chirurgical de L'Hallux varus iatrogénique. Med Chir Pied 1991;7:9–16.
12. Lau JT, Myerson MS. Modified split extensor hallucis longus tendon transfer for correction of hallux varus. Foot Ankle Int 2002;23(12):1138–40.
13. Myerson MS, Komenda GA. Results of hallux varus correction using an extensor hallucis brevis tenodesis. Foot Ankle Int 1996;17:21–7.
14. Skalley TC, Myerson MS. The operative treatment of acquired hallux varus. Clin Orthop Relat Res 1994;306:183–91.

15. Gerbert J, Traynor C, Blue K, et al. Use of the Mini TightRope® for correction of hallux varus deformity. J Foot Ankle Surg 2011;50(2):245–51.

16. Plovanich EJ, Donnenwerth MP, Abicht BP, et al. Failure after soft-tissue release with tendon transfer for flexible iatrogenic hallux varus: a systematic review. J Foot Ankle Surg 2012;51(2):195–7.

Soft Tissue Balancing After Partial Foot Amputations

Caitlin S. Garwood, DPM[a], John S. Steinberg, DPM[b,c,*]

KEYWORDS

- Transmetatarsal amputation • Lisfranc amputation • Chopart amputation
- Tibialis anterior • Tendo-Achilles lengthening

KEY POINTS

- Partial foot amputations can have successful outcomes if appropriate soft tissue balancing procedures are performed to address equinus and varus deformities that develop.
- Transmetatarsal amputations (TMAs), Lisfranc amputations, and Chopart amputations often require tendo-Achilles lengthening (TAL) procedures to address the equinus deformity that frequently develops from the overpowering of the gastrocnemius-soleus complex.
- A varus deformity can be addressed after partial foot amputation with an anterior tibial tendon lengthening, anterior tibial tendon transfer, or other adjunctive soft tissue procedure.

INTRODUCTION

Despite consistent advances in medicine and surgery, limb loss continues to be prevalent in society. Every year an estimated 185,000 new amputations of the lower extremity are performed in the United States.[1] It has been predicted that by 2050 the number of people living with limb loss will more than double to 3.6 million.[2] It was previously thought that a major amputation, including below-knee amputation or above-knee amputation, was preferable to a partial foot amputation. Partial foot amputations, however, maintain a full length, functional extremity that often requires only a foot orthosis, bracing, or toe filler compared with a full lower-extremity prostheses. Partial foot amputations also carry a decreased mortality and decreased energy expenditure compared with proximal limb loss amputations.[3–5] Partial foot amputations are now

[a] Department of Plastic Surgery, Center for Wound Healing and Hyperbaric Medicine, MedStar Georgetown University Hospital, 3800 Reservoir Road, Northwest, Washington, DC 20007, USA;
[b] Department of Plastic Surgery, Center for Wound Healing and Hyperbaric Medicine, MedStar Georgetown University Hospital, Georgetown University School of Medicine, 3800 Reservoir Road, Northwest, Washington, DC 20007, USA; [c] Podiatric Residency Program, MedStar Washington Hospital Center, 110 Irving Street, Northwest, Washington, DC 20010, USA
* Corresponding author. Department of Plastic Surgery, Center for Wound Healing and Hyperbaric Medicine, MedStar Georgetown University Hospital, 3800 Reservoir Road, Northwest, Washington, DC 20007.
E-mail address: jss5@gunet.georgetown.edu

Clin Podiatr Med Surg 33 (2016) 99–111
http://dx.doi.org/10.1016/j.cpm.2015.06.005
0891-8422/16/$ – see front matter © 2016 Elsevier Inc. All rights reserved.

the most common type of amputation and are estimated to occur almost twice as frequently as major amputations. A majority of these amputations are due to diabetes, peripheral vascular disease, or trauma.[2] The outcomes of any type of amputation can have a major physical and mental impact on patients and forever change their lives. It is imperative to recognize this impact to appropriately and efficiently heal patients after amputation and prevent future complications.

Partial foot amputations are highly technique-dependent procedures and when done appropriately can have excellent outcomes. Too often, there is a belief that partial foot amputations and limb salvage procedures are basic and easy. This is an unfortunate misconception because there are many complex factors affecting the outcome and longevity of amputations. Surgeons must consider the numerous comorbidities that these patients often present with, including diabetes, cardiovascular disease, renal disease, peripheral vascular disease, and malnutrition. They must also consider the rehabilitation of patients and their ability to ambulate with their residual limb. The need for a functional outcome can often assist in decision making for the appropriate level of amputation that is to be performed. Perhaps the greatest complication associated with partial foot amputations is the development of equinus and equinovarus deformities, which can lead to reulceration, breakdown, or complete failure. Because of these complications, foot and ankle surgeons must consider the biomechanics of partial foot amputations and the potential need for tendon balancing procedures.[6]

Most partial foot amputations only involve the digits or metatarsophalangeal joints (MTPJs) but approximately 24% are at the transmetatarsal level or more proximal.[1,7] With digital and MTPJ amputations, there are only minor imbalances seen because most still maintain a majority of tendon insertions to the foot. With transmetatarsal, Lisfranc, and Chopart amputations, however, the development of structural and biomechanical deformities is often seen because these amputations involve a significant loss of tendon insertions as well as other important soft tissue structures. Several structures can be addressed with lengthening procedures or tendon transfers, including the gastrocnemius-soleus complex, the anterior tibial tendon, and the peroneal tendons. The appropriate selection and timing of procedure can help maintain a functioning limb and reduce future complications.

SURGICAL PLANNING

Appropriate surgical planning and decision making is an imperative step for both surgeon and patient when considering partial foot amputations. Planning must always begin with a detailed evaluation of the patient as well as the foot.

One of the most important aspects of surgical planning is assessing the patient's goals. It is crucial to understand if a patient is ambulatory preoperatively or not. If a patient is not ambulatory, then a partial foot amputation may not be the best option, especially if there is any belief that it will not heal. Younger and more active patients are often more successful with a below-knee amputation given the advanced functional capacity delivered through recent advances in prosthetics.

Medical optimization should always be performed prior to amputation. Comorbidities, including diabetes, chronic renal failure, peripheral vascular disease, and malnutrition, can have detrimental effects on the success and healing of amputations. Prior to surgical intervention, a cohesive and complete multidisciplinary team should be consulted for care of the patient. The team approach includes internal medicine, endocrinology, infectious disease, podiatric surgery, vascular surgery, plastic surgery, orthopedic surgery, nephrology, dieticians, prosthetists and other specialists when necessary. The overall outcome for a patient depends on foverall health and functional ability.

Vascular status is one of the most important factors to consider when determining the level of amputation. The incision placement must be made in an area of adequate blood flow to allow for healing of the amputation site. A full vascular evaluation should be performed, including pulse examination with a handheld Doppler, ankle and toe brachial indices, and a vascular consult when necessary. The vascular consult helps determine if any revascularization procedure needs to be performed prior to final amputation, closure, or adjunctive soft tissue procedures. It is important to evaluate the vascular status prior to performing any soft tissue balancing procedures that create new incisions and potential for nonhealing.

Preoperatively it is important to evaluate the patient's foot structure and any potential for deformities that may occur postoperatively. For example, the ankle range of motion (ROM) should be assessed to determine if there is a preexisting equinus deformity. This should be assessed this by dorsiflexing the ankle with the knee bent as well as with the knee extended. A lack of 10° of dorsiflexion indicates an ankle equinus deformity. This is extremely important because there is a loss of power across the ankle during gait once the metatarsal heads have been compromised.[8–10] After a TMA, the ipsilateral ankle can only use 70% of the static ROM available compared with 90% on an unaffected ankle.[8] The timing of soft tissue balancing procedures often depends on the surgeon and the surgeon experience. It is an emerging standard of care that a TAL should be performed on all patients receiving a partial foot amputation that exhibit an equinus deformity. Most surgeons perform this procedure at the time of definitive closure of the amputation site. Many of the other adjunctive procedures can be performed at this same definitive procedure if the physician thinks they will prevent future breakdown. They can also be easily performed, however, as outpatient procedures during the follow-up period if a patient begins to exhibit an equinus or varus deformity or begins to develop signs of increased pressure areas at the amputation site.

TRANSMETATARSAL AMPUTATION

The TMA was first introduced in 1855 by Bernard and Heute for a patient with trench foot, but it was not until 1949 that McKittrick and colleagues[11] used this amputation for management of diabetic foot ulcers and gangrene.[12] The healing rates after TMA vary greatly in the literature, from 44% to 92%.[11,13,14] Patients undergoing TMA have a higher revision rate than more proximal amputations, with rates of 30% to 40% in diabetic and vascular patients.[14–19] Despite the success and utility of the TMA, several factors must be considered and addressed to avoid the development of equinus or equinovarus. These deformities can cause prolonged nonhealing, new ulceration, or breakdown of the amputation incision. New ulcerations and breakdown are most often seen at the plantar-distal amputation or along the plantar-lateral foot.

When a TMA is performed, it is up to the surgeon to determine the level at which the metatarsal bones are transected. This is often determined by the vascular status, soft tissue coverage, and extent of infection. It is ideal to maintain as much metatarsal length as possible to maintain a normal transverse and longitudinal arch of the foot.[20] Through the course of the amputation several tendon insertions are sacrificed, including the extensor hallucis longus (EHL), extensor digitorum longus (EDL), and sometimes the peroneus tertius. Occasionally the peroneus brevis may be affected as well, depending on the proximity of the osteotomies in the metatarsal shafts. It is recommended to mark out the bases of the first and fifth metatarsals to avoid sacrificing the insertions of the tibialis anterior and peroneus brevis tendons. It is the loss of these tendon insertions that exaggerates the imbalance of the partial foot amputation.

After amputation, the tibialis anterior remains intact as the only ankle dorsiflexor. The gastrocnemius-soleus complex greatly overpowers the tibialis anterior, leading to an equinus deformity. When left untreated, this creates an increased plantar pressure on the remaining forefoot and amputation stump.[21–23] The tibialis anterior and posterior are strong invertors of the foot and tend to overpower the evertors of the foot, the peroneus brevis and peroneus longus. This can result in a varus position of the rearfoot, which can lead to increased pressure on the plantar-lateral aspect of the residual limb. The effect on the intrinsic muscles and plantar fascia insertion must also be considered. This has been described as a loss of a rigid beam effect, causing increased plantar stump pressure, exaggerated varus, and subtalar joint imbalance.[24,25]

To address the deformities that are present after a TMA, several tendon balancing procedures have been described. The gastrocnemius-soleus complex is the most important structure to address and also the most frequently addressed consistently by foot and ankle surgeons by lengthening the tendon. Because the tibialis anterior can be a deforming force, this can be addressed through lengthening or transfer procedures. Other tendons that have been considered for balancing include the peroneus longus and peroneus brevis, the flexor hallucis longus (FHL), and the EDL.

LISFRANC AMPUTATION

Although a TMA is the most common and preferable partial foot amputation to perform, a Lisfranc amputation should be considered when there is more extensive soft tissue loss, infection, or vascular compromise. Lisfranc amputations can be successful in properly selected patients with the properly selected adjunctive procedures. It is performed at the level of the tarsometatarsal joint and all of the metatarsals are removed. The biggest downside of this partial foot amputation is the effect on specific musculo-tendinous structures. The tibialis anterior, peroneus brevis, and peroneus tertius insertions are sacrificed during a Lisfranc amputation. This leads to an overpowering of the posterior tibial tendon as well as the gastrocnemius-soleus complex, leading to equino-varus.[26] To avoid the inevitable equinovarus deformity, it is recommended to maintain the base of the first and fifth metatarsals if at all possible.[20] If the insertions are completely sacrificed, then soft tissue balancing procedures should be performed.

Similar to a TMA, there is a loss of major dorsiflexors, including tibialis anterior, EHL, and EDL, which leads to an overpowering of the tendo-Achilles. For this reason, it is customary to perform a TAL procedure (described later). The choice of lengthening in this instance should be a percutaneous TAL, gastrocnemius recession, tenotomy, or tenectomy. The decision is largely surgeon driven and the complications of over-lengthening versus the effects of under-lengthening must be considered.

CHOPART AMPUTATION

Chopart amputations were introduced by Francois Chopart in 1792, as he described an amputation at the talonavicular and calcaneocuboid joints.[27] It was originally not seen as a favorable amputation due to the frequent ulceration and breakdown distally. Over the past 100 years, many osseous and tendinous procedures have been attempted to prevent equinovarus and distal breakdown. Regardless of the procedure and tendon balancing, success of Chopart amputations often relies on postoperative accommodation and bracing.[27,28] A systematic review looked at the literature associated with success of Chopart amputations and concluded that despite the osseous or tendinous procedures performed, a functional limb can be achieved with appropriate high-profile prosthetics. They also saw that most complications or breakdowns occurred with ill-fitting devices or with unprotected ambulation.[27]

Because of loss of the extensor muscles with a Chopart amputation, a TAL procedure is pivotal. The procedure of choice for the authors is an Achilles tenectomy where a 1- to 2-cm portion of the tendon is removed to prevent reattachment of the tenotomy (discussed later). This allows for the most aggressive release of the tendon and prevents recurrence. The functionality in this instance is not as important because the patient requires lifelong bracing and prosthetics.

Other procedures include anchoring the anterior tibial tendon into the neck of the talus.[28] This was first described to combat the equinus pull of the Achilles tendon. This requires anchoring the tendon into the talus, which introduces a foreign substance into the wound and also potential for rupture or breakdown at the site. Similarly, the extensor tendons or the posterior tibial tendons can be transferred to the talus.[29] In complex medical patients, these procedures are often not recommended because the benefits often do not outweigh the risks. As discussed previously, the patients will be in a lifelong prosthetic for protection as well.

ANKLE AND SUBTALAR ARTHRODESIS

Due to the severe equinus deformity that often occurs after Chopart amputations, 2 techniques have been utilized to perform an ankle and subtalar joint fusion to obtain a functional limb.[29,30] Persson and Soderberg[30] described their technique as it was performed on 2 patients using staples at the fusion sites. DeGere and Grady[29] described their technique using an intramedullary nail through the calcaneus and talus and into the tibia. This procedure was performed on 7 patients. At 1 year there was no reculceration or stump breakdown and all had a rigid rearfoot without equinovarus. Patients were either ambulating with a patellar tendon brace, a clamshell prosthesis, or a modified cast boot.[29] Although there are few data on this technique, it could prove useful in the properly selected patient. The biggest drawbacks are that it introduces a large amount of hardware, increasing the risk of infection, and requires major additional dissection and surgery.

GASTROCNEMIUS-SOLEUS COMPLEX

The gastrocnemius-soleus complex is almost always addressed when performing a partial foot amputation. Not only does a partial foot amputation often lead to an equinus deformity but also many patients have a preexisting equinus present. This is especially prevalent in diabetic patients who have been shown to have increased density of collagen fibrils within the Achilles tendon that leads to stiffness and lack of motion.[31,32] It is also well established that an equinus contracture leads to increased plantar pressures, which increases the risk of ulceration or failure of partial foot amputation.[32–38] Correcting and preventing this deformity can increase the success of these amputations and allow for a better functional result. Gastrocnemius recession, percutaneous teno-Achilles lengthening, and tenotomy/tenectomy are the 3 main surgical options that exist, and each has its own indications, advantages, and disadvantages (**Table 1**). Proper selection of procedure is important to ensure the best outcomes.

Percutaneous Tendo-Achilles Lengthening

The percutaneous TAL is the authors' frequent procedure of choice after a TMA and often after a Lisfranc amputation. The use of the TAL after partial foot amputation significantly weakens the posterior musculature in hopes of reducing pressure at the amputation site. It is also advantageous to use this technique in patients with peripheral vascular disease because it leaves minimal incisions for healing.[37] Barry and colleagues[15] performed 33 TAL procedures for treatment of chronic ulcerations after

Table 1
Comparison of gastrocnemius recession, tendo-Achilles lengthening, and tenectomy/tenotomy for lengthening of the gastrocnemius-soleus complex for equinus deformity associated with partial foot amputation

Procedure	Indications	Advantage	Disadvantage
Gastrocnemius recession	• Mild or moderate equinus	• Decreased risk of over-lengthening or calcaneal gait • Decreased risk of Achilles rupture • Can weight bear	• Inadequate lengthening • Larger incision
TAL	• Moderate to severe equinus	• Percutaneous • Can be done in peripheral vascular disease patients	• Postoperative NWB • Calcaneal gait • Over-lengthening • Achilles rupture
Tenectomy or tenotomy	• Severe equinus	• Large correction • Low risk of recurrence	• Postoperative NWB • Calcaneal gait • Over-lengthening

TMA. They saw a 91% healing rate of the ulcerations. Attinger and colleagues[20] saw a reduction in late transmetatarsal reulceration rate from 50% to 4% after performing TALs. La Fontaine and colleagues[22] found, however, that 16 of 28 patients who had a TMA developed a new or recurrent ulceration despite having a TAL, demonstrating that other factors may need to be addressed as well.

The surgical technique that is typically used by the authors is the triple hemisection as described by Hoke[39] and is demonstrated in **Fig. 1**. It can be performed with the patient in the supine position. The superior aspect of the calcaneus is palpated and marked off with a skin marker. A ruler is then used to measure 3 cm, 6 cm, and 9 cm proximal to the palpable superior aspect of the calcaneus. The medial and lateral aspects of the Achilles tendon are palpated and a 15 blade is then used to make a small incision through the skin in the most distal incision site. The tendon is then cut from the central aspect of the tendon through the medial aspect, being sure to only transect approximately 50% of the tendon. The same thing is performed with the remaining 2 incisions, with the middle hemisection occurring on the lateral 50% of the tendon and the proximal incision on the medial 50%. This can be performed similarly with 2 hemisections laterally and the middle hemisection medially depending on surgeon preference. During the procedure, someone is to hold the leg while applying a gentle dorsiflexion at the ankle. A gentle give should be felt with each hemisection.

The risks associated with percutaneous TAL are tendon rupture, loss of plantar-flexory strength, and over-lengthening of the tendon, which can lead to calcaneal gait. In 2006, Mohsen Allam[40] reported calcaneal gait with a heel ulceration in 16.7% of patients undergoing TAL and TMA. Calcaneal gait has the potential for devastating outcomes, including a more proximal amputation, and the surgeon must take extra care in ensuring adequate Achilles lengthening without over-lengthening.

Gastrocnemius Recession

The gastrocnemius recession is typically indicated for mild to moderate ankle equinus. It is used more often for flat foot reconstruction or cerebral palsy, but it is an option after partial foot amputation as well.[28] It has been described for patients who have only a gastrocnemius equinus deformity because it does not sacrifice the soleus

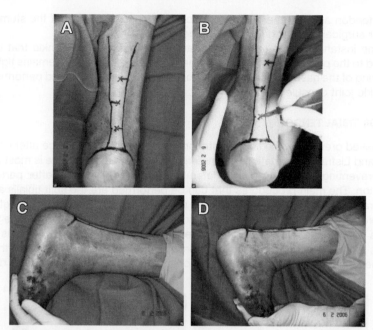

Fig. 1. Percutaneous tendo-Achilles lengthening procedure. (*A*) Superior aspect of the calcaneus is marked and incisions are marked at 3 cm, 6 cm, and 9 cm proximal. (*B*) A 15 blade is used to complete the hemisections. (*C*) Preoperative assessment of ankle dorsiflexion. (*D*) Postoperative assessment of ankle dorsiflexion showing significant increase dorsiflexion.

muscle. It has been seen to have a more controlled lengthening and, therefore, decreases the risk of over-lengthening and the potential for calcaneal gait.[32,34]

Disadvantages are that it requires a larger incision placed on the calf that could have a potential for nonhealing, especially in diabetic and peripheral vascular patients who are often receiving these partial foot amputations. It also has the potential to inadequately restore ankle motion with increased incidence of ankle equinus recurrence. There is an increased risk of nerve injury due to the close proximity of the sural nerve as well as more scar-related issues postoperatively.[32,34,37]

The technique that can be used most easily and most often is the Strayer, where a transverse sectioning of the gastrocnemius aponeurosis is performed.[41] Some surgeons prefer a Vulpius- or Baker-type procedure that uses either a chevron or tongue-in-groove recession.[42,43] It is mostly surgeon preference when deciding which procedure to perform but some functioning of the gastrocnemius remains with the Vulpius or Baker. The gastrocnemius recession is less frequently performed after partial foot amputation because it is typically seen as inadequate.

Tenotomy/Tenectomy

The final option discussed is an Achilles tenotomy or tenectomy. This is the most aggressive TAL option and is the procedure of choice for the authors when performing a Chopart amputation. A tenotomy is a complete transection of the Achilles tendon and a tenectomy involves removal of approximately 1 cm of the transected tendon.[32] An Achilles lengthening or tenotomy is often deemed inadequate for Chopart amputation and the authors think that a tenectomy best reduces the unopposed pull of the

Achilles tendon and has the best chance of preventing ulceration of the stump (See **Fig. 2** for surgical approach to Achilles tenectomy.)

In some instances there remains contracture deformity at the ankle that can be attributed to the posterior joint capsule. If the posterior joint capsule remains tight after lengthening of the gastrocnemius-soleus complex, the surgeon should perform a posterior ankle joint capsule release.

ANTERIOR TIBIAL TENDON

As discussed previously, the tibialis anterior is a major deforming force after transmetatarsal and Lisfranc amputations. An anterior tibial tendon procedure is most beneficial in preventing or healing plantar-lateral ulcerations that occur after partial foot amputation. The main procedures that can be performed are the split tibialis anterior tendon transfer (STATT), a complete tibialis anterior tendon transfer, and a lengthening procedure. There are advantages and disadvantages of each procedure. The tendon transfers require 3 additional incisions whereas the lengthening only involves 1. The transfers rely on good bone quality to appropriately anchor the tendon into the midfoot. When transferring a tendon, the surgeon must also get the exact tension desired;

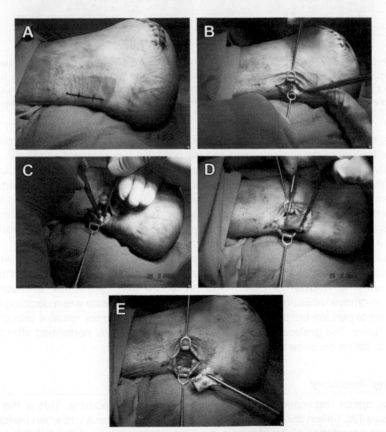

Fig. 2. Achilles tenectomy. (*A*) A 2-cm incision along the lateral aspect of the Achilles tendon. (*B*) Dissection performed through the paratenon to clearly identify the tendon. (*C*, *D*) The tendon is transected distally and brought through the incision to expose the proximal portion. (*E*) A 1-cm section is then removed from the distal portion of the cut tendon.

otherwise; there may be under- or over-correction of the deformity. Similarly, a simple lengthening procedure could leave the patient with residual varus deformity by inadequate lengthening.

When performing a tendon transfer, whether STATT or complete, a 3-incision approach is most commonly used. The first incision is made over the insertion point of the tendon along the dorsal-medial aspect of the first metatarsal-cuneiform joint. The second incision is made along the anterior aspect of the lower leg above the ankle joint and along the anterior tibial tendon. The anterior tibial tendon is carefully dissected free from its most distal insertion and pulled through the proximal incision. If transferring only half the tendon, then dissect free only the lateral portion of the tendon. The third incision is made over the dorsal aspect of the lateral cuneiform or the cuboid and dissected to the level of bone. Intraoperative fluoroscopy can be used to ensure adequate incision placement for this. The tibialis anterior is then routed into the third incision, being sure to stay underneath the extensor retinaculum.[44] The tendon is then fixated using a biotenodesis screw, buttonhole technique, or tendon anchors.[25] Appropriate tension must be achieved prior to final fixation. This technique is challenging because patients with partial foot amputations often have poor soft tissue envelopes, poor bone quality, poor vascular supply, and already weakened tendons.

Similar to a TAL, the anterior tibial lengthening effectively weakens the pull of the muscle to alleviate the varus deformity. The anterior tibial lengthening is performed through a 1-incision approach. The anterior tibial tendon is palpated along the anterior aspect of the lower leg and a 2- to 3-cm incision is placed along the tendon just above the level of the ankle joint. Dissection is carried to the level of the tendon and a small incision is made through the tendon sheath. Once clearly identified, a Z-type lengthening is performed in the tendon with 2 hemisections in the tendon, being sure to leave adequate tendon length between the hemisections. The tendon is then stretched to lengthen as necessary. This method is currently the method of choice for the authors because it adequately alleviates pressure on the plantar-lateral aspect of the foot and has a decreased incidence of any major complications in a high-risk patient population. The most success has been seen with ulcerations that occur on the plantar-lateral aspect of the foot distal to the Lisfranc joint.

PERONEAL TENDONS

The peroneus longus and peroneus brevis muscles are important structures to consider in functionality of partial foot amputations. The peroneus brevis is sacrificed during a Lisfranc or Chopart amputation and sometimes for a TMA. The peroneus longus is sacrificed for a Chopart amputation and partially for a Lisfranc. When the peroneus brevis insertion is lost during amputation, one of the major evertors of the foot is lost. As discussed previously, the partial foot is often then overpowered by the invertors and a varus deformity develops. Some procedures have been developed to try to compensate for this and to maintain the strength of the peroneus brevis.

Schweinberger and Roukis[45] first described a balancing procedure for the TMA using a peroneus brevis to peroneus longus tendon transfer. They believe that this transfer can assist with plantarflexing the first ray as well as everting the forefoot. Their technique describes an incision from the tip of the fibula to the fifth metatarsal base. They then detach the peroneus brevis from its insertion and weave it through the peroneus longus. After appropriate tension is applied, ensuring the foot is no longer in a varus position, the tendons are sutured together. Patients must remain non–weight bearing (NWB) for 4 to 6 weeks. They looked at 7 patients, 9 feet, who underwent a peroneus brevis to peroneus longus transfer. They saw that all patients had adequate correction of the varus deformity with no recurrent or new forefoot ulcerations noted at 14.6 months. Some of the disadvantages are the need to heal another incision, need for NWB, and tendon rupture.[35]

Other procedures include anchoring the peroneus brevis into the cuboid or the lateral aspect of the foot. This can be performed at the time of the amputation and could eliminate the need for a secondary incision. If performed after the amputation, then a small incision is required at the level of the cuboid and fifth metatarsal base. The difficulty with this procedure is identifying and obtaining a sufficient amount and length of the peroneus brevis tendon to adequately anchor it into the cuboid. It can be anchored by a trephine bone plug, a biotenodesis screw, the buttonhole technique, or tunnels.[25] Potential complications are similar but this often involves the introduction of a foreign material, because the most common type of fixation today is the biotenodesis screw. Often in the complex patient population, difficulty is found with the patient's bone stock and obtaining appropriate fixation of the tendon. Schweinberger and Roukis[35] described a method of peroneus brevis and anterior tibial tendon transfer by using trephine bone plugs into the cuboid and medial cuneiform. They frequently perform this on amputations at the level of the Lisfranc joint.[35]

OTHER PROCEDURES

Besides the procedures discussed previously, there are a few other procedures that have been performed to balance the foot after partial foot amputation. Attinger and colleagues[20] discuss tenodesis of the flexor and extensor tendons from the fourth and fifth toes with the foot held in neutral. The theory is that it is relatively simple, can be done at the time of the amputation, and may oppose some of the potential for varus. Some investigators believe, however, that this leaves dysvascular structures in the wound bed, which could lead to a higher likelihood of failure and it also may not be strong enough to completely oppose the strength of the tibialis anterior or gastrocnemius-soleus complex.[35]

The final procedure worth mentioning is transfer of the FHL and EDL tendons for a TMA, as described by Roukis.[46] The technique involves anchoring the FHL tendon through a drill hole in the first metatarsal from plantar to dorsal and the EDL tendon into the fourth metatarsal. It is advantageous because it uses tendons that have already been sacrificed during the amputation. The theory is that it allows for plantarflexion and eversion of the medial column in conjunction with dorsiflexion and eversion of the lateral column.[46] Disadvantages involve the introduction of foreign material, potential for metatarsal fracture, and potential for poor bone quality.

COMPLICATIONS

All surgical procedures have potential for complications. A majority of partial foot amputations are occurring in diabetic or peripheral vascular patients where the complication rates are inherently higher. As with any surgical procedure, patients could experience infection, wound dehiscence, pain, swelling, blood clot, change in gait and function, and many others including ischemia, nonhealing, and delayed healing.[6] Soft tissue balancing procedures pose their own set of unique complications.

There is potential for over- or under-lengthening of a tendon or improper tensioning. This could lead to new or worse complications, such as calcaneal gait after an over-lengthened TAL. This has been reported to occur in 16.7% of patients undergoing a TMA with TAL.[40] Under-lengthening can lead to recurrent or continued ulceration or failure of the amputation. Similarly, improper tensioning can lead to failure of the procedure due to over- or under-correction of the deformity.

After lengthening or transferring a tendon, the tendon is weakened. This can cause a tendon rupture if the tendon is not offloaded adequately or the patient is unable to remain NWB. For example, the TAL is often performed in the watershed area of the Achilles; thus, there is an increased risk of tendon rupture after lengthening. Tendon procedures can also cause dysfunction or weakness in the tendon. In 1 study, 80% of patients reported persistent stiffness and 38% reported weakness after TAL.[47]

Even though these procedures are aimed at preventing or eliminating new and recurrent ulcerations, there is still a risk of them developing. A study by La Fontaine and colleagues[22] looked at the rate of new and recurrent ulcerations in patients who had a TMA with TAL performed. They reported a 35% recurrence rate of ulcerations, and 6 of 28 patients developed an ulcer in a new location. This led to 57% of the patients having a new or recurrent ulceration after TMA with TAL at a mean follow-up of 2.4 years.[22]

POSTOPERATIVE CARE

For most of the procedures discussed previously, patients are recommended to remain NWB in an off-loading posterior splint or walking boot. The length of NWB often depends on the healing of the amputation site. If, for example a TAL was performed in conjunction to a TMA closure, then the patient remains NWB until the amputation site is completely healed. It is often difficult for many of these patients to remain entirely NWB; thus, appropriate protection with a boot or splint must be in place at all times to avoid any potential rupture of the tendon. If the procedure is performed separately from the amputation, then they are to remain NWB for approximately 4 weeks to allow for proper tendon healing. It is imperative in the postoperative period that patients be fit for appropriate shoes or shoes fillers to adequately protect the extremity prior to initiation of full ambulation.

SUMMARY

Partial foot amputations can have successful outcomes and are critical procedures for the limb salvage surgeon. The goal should be to obtain a well-balanced plantigrade foot that has the least potential for future breakdown. The equinus and varus deformities that often occur with these amputations must be addressed. There are several surgical procedures that can be performed to balance and offload high-pressure areas. Some of the most beneficial procedures performed are the TAL and the tibialis anterior tendon transfer or lengthening. Proper surgical planning must be used to appropriately address any deformity and give each patient the best potential to heal and remain healed.

REFERENCES

1. Owings M, Kozak L. Ambulatory and inpatient procedures in the United States, 1996. Vital Health Stat 13 1998;139:1–119.
2. Ziegler-Graham K, MacKenzie EJ, Ephraim PL, et al. Estimating the prevalence of limb loss in the United States: 2005 to 2050. Arch Phys Med Rehabil 2008;89: 422–9.
3. Waters RL, Perry J, Antonelli D, et al. Energy cost of walking of amputees: the influence of level of amputation. J Bone Joint Surg Am 1976;58:42–6.

4. Pinzur MS, Gold J, Schwartz D, et al. Energy demands for walking in dysvascular amputees as related to the level of amputation. Orthopaedics 1993;15: 1033–73.
5. Harris KA, van Schie L, Carroll SE, et al. Rehabilitation potential of elderly patients with major amputations. J Cardiovasc Surg 1991;32:463–7.
6. Sullivan JP. Complications of pedal amputations. Clin Podiatr Med Surg 2005;22: 4469–84.
7. Dillingham T, Pezzin L, MacKenzie E. Limb amputaions and limb deficiency: epidemiology and recent trends in the United States. South Med J 2002;95: 875–83.
8. Tang SF, Chen CP, Chen MJ. Transmetatarsal amputation prosthesis with carbon-fiber plate: enhanced gait function. Am J Phys Med Rehabil 2004;83:124–30.
9. Garbalosa J, Cavanagh P, Wu G, et al. Foot function in the diabetic patients after partial amputation. Foot Ankle Int 1996;17:43–8.
10. Mueller MJ, Salisch GB, Bastian AJ. Differences in the gait characteristics of people with diabetes and transmetatarsal amputation compared with age-matched controls. Gait Posture 1998;7:200–6.
11. McKittrick LS, McKittrick JB, Risley TS. Transmetatarsal amputation for infection or gangrene in patients with diabetes mellitus. Ann Surg 1949;130:826–42.
12. Schwindt CD, Lulloff RS, Rogers SC. Transmetatarsal amputations. Orthop Clin North Am 1973;4:31–42.
13. Hodge MJ, Peters TG, Efird WG. Amputation of the distal portion of the foot. South Med J 1989;82:1138–42.
14. Hosch J, Quiroga C, Bosma J, et al. Outcomes of transmetatarsal amputations in patients with diabetes mellitus. J Foot Ankle Surg 1997;36(6):430–4.
15. Barry DC, Sabacinski KA, Habershaw GM, et al. Tendo Achillis procedures for chronic ulcerations in diabetic patients with transmetatarsal amputations. J Am Podiatr Med Assoc 1993;83:96–100.
16. Dalla Paola L, Faglia E, Caminiti M, et al. Ulcer recurrence following first ray amputation in diabetic patients:a cohort prospective study. Diabetes Care 2003;26:1874–8.
17. Rosenblum BI, Freeman DV. Surgical revision of the problematic transmetatarsal amputation. J Am Podiatr Med Assoc 1993;83:91–5.
18. Larsson V, Anderson G. Partial amputation of the foot for diabetic or arteriosclerotic gangrene. J Bone Joint Surg Br 1978;60:126–30.
19. Wallace GF, Stapleton JJ. Transmetatarsal amputations. Clin Podiatr Med Surg 2005;22:365–84.
20. Attinger C, Venturi M, Kim K, et al. Maximizing the length and optimizing biomechanics in foot amputations by avoiding cookbook recipes for amputation. Semin Vasc Surg 2003;16(1):44–66.
21. Aronow MS, Diaz-Doran V, Sullivan RJ, et al. The effect of triceps surae contracture force on plantar foot pressure distribution. Foot Ankle Int 2006;27:43–52.
22. La Fontaine J, Brown D, Adams M, et al. New and recurrent ulcerations after percutaneous Achilles tendon lengthening in transmetatarsal amputation. J Foot Ankle Surg 2008;47(3):225–9.
23. Van Gils CC, Roeder B. The effect of ankle equinus upon the diabetic foot. Clin Podiatr Med Surg 2002;19:391–409.
24. Chrzan J, Giurini J. A biomechanical model for the transmetatarsal amputation. J Am Podiatr Med Assoc 1993;83:82–6.
25. Clark GD, Lui E, Cook KD. Tendon balancing in pedal amputations. Clin Podiatr Med Surg 2005;22(3):447–67.

26. DeCotiis MA. Lisfranc and Chopart amputations. Clin Podiatr Med Surg 2005;22: 385–93.
27. Schade VL, Roukis TS, Yan JL. Factors associated with successful Chopart amputation in patients with diabetes. Foot Ankle Spec 2010;3(5):278–84.
28. Reyzelman AM, Hadi S, Armstrong DG. Limb salvage with Chopart's amputation and tendon balancing. J Am Podiatr Med Assoc 1999;89(2):100–3.
29. DeGere MW, Grady JF. A modification of Chopart's amputation with ankle and subtalar arthrodesis by using an intramedullary nail. J Foot Ankle Surg 2005;44(4):281–6.
30. Persson BM, Soderberg B. Pantalar fusion for correction of painful equinus after traumatic Chopart's amputation: a report of 2 cases. Acta Orthop Scand 1996;67:300–2.
31. Grant WP, Sullivan R, Sonenshine DE, et al. Electron microscopic investigation of the effects of diabetes mellitus on the Achilles tendon. J Foot Ankle Surg 1997; 36(4):272–8.
32. Greenhagen RM, Johnson AR, Bevilacqua NJ. Gastrocnemius recession or tendo-achilles lengthening for equinus deformity in the diabetic foot. Clin Podiatr Med Surg 2012;29:413–24.
33. Lavery LA, Armstrong DG, Boulton AJ. Ankle equinus deformity and its relationship to high plantar pressure in a large population with diabetes mellitus. J Am Podiatr Med Assoc 2002;92(9):479–82.
34. Nishimoto GS, Attinger CE, Cooper PS. Lengthening the Achilles tendon for the treatment of diabetic plantar forefoot ulceration. Surg Clin North Am 2003; 83(3):707–26.
35. Schweinberger MH, Roukis TS. Soft tissue and osseous techniques to balance forefoot and midfoot amputations. Clin Podiatr Med Surg 2008;25:623–39.
36. Armstrong D, Stacpoole-Shea S, Nguyen H, et al. Lengthening of the achilles tendon in diabetic patients who are at high risk for ulceration of the foot. J Bone Joint Surg Am 1999;81:535–8.
37. Schweinberger MH, Roukis TS. Surgical correction of soft-tissue ankle equines contracture. Clin Podiatr Med Surg 2008;25:571–85.
38. Mueller M, Sinacore D, Hastings M, et al. Effect of Achilles tendon lengthening on neuropathic plantar ulcers. J Bone Joint Surg Am 2003;85:1436 45.
39. Hoke M. An operation for the correction of extremely relaxed flat feet. J Bone Joint Surg 1931;13:773–83.
40. Mohsen Allam A. Impact of Achilles tendon lengthening (ATL) on the diabetic plantar forefoot ulceration. Egypt J Plast Reconstr Surg 2006;30(1):43–8.
41. Strayer LM Jr. Recession of the gastrocnemius; an operation to relieve spastic contracture of the calf muscles. J Bone Joint Surg Am 1950;32(3):671–6.
42. Vulpius O, Stoffel A. Tenotomie der end schnen der mm. Gastrocnemius el soleus mittels mittels rutschenlassen nach Vulpius. In: Ferdinard Enke, editor. Orthopadische Operationslehre. Stuttgart (Germany): Nabu Press; 1913. p. 29–31.
43. Baker LD. A rational approach to the surgical needs of the cerebral palsy patient. J Bone Joint Surg Am 1956;38(2):313–23.
44. Southerland JT, Boberg JS, Downey MS, et al. McGlamry's comprehensive textbook of foot and ankle surgery. 4th edition. Philadelphia: LWW; 2013.
45. Schweinberger MH, Roukis TS. Balancing of the transmetatarsal amputation with peroneus brevis to longus tendon transfer. J Foot Ankle Surg 2007;46(6):510–4.
46. Roukis TS. Flexor hallucis longus and extensor digitorum longus tendon transfers for balancing the foot following transmetatarsal amputation. J Foot Ankle Surg 2009;48(3):398–401.
47. Stauff MP, Kilgore WB, Joyner PW, et al. Functional outcome after percutaneous tendo-Achilles lengthening. Foot Ankle Surg 2010;17(1):29–32.

Flexor Hallucis Longus Tendon Transfer for Calcific Insertional Achilles Tendinopathy

Michael A. Howell, DPM, Alan R. Catanzariti, DPM*

KEYWORDS

- Achilles tendonitis • Flexor hallucis longus tendon transfer • Insertional calcification
- Insertional tendinosis • Retrocalcaneal bursitis

KEY POINTS

- Calcific insertional Achilles tendinitis or tendinopathy (CIAT) is a common musculoskeletal condition that can result in significant pain and disability.
- There is limited evidence-based support for the current therapeutic interventions used to treat CIAT.
- Nonoperative therapy is unsuccessful in 24% to 45.5% of patients with CIAT.
- Surgery for CIAT should be considered in patients with refractory disease, persistent pain, and significant disability.
- Surgical management for CIAT should be comprehensive, addressing all pathologic components of the disease process.
- This article describes the authors' approach to surgical management of CIAT.

Video of surgical technique for the treatment of CIAT with FHL tendon transfer accompanies this article at http://www.podiatric.theclinics.com/

INTRODUCTION

Calcific insertional Achilles tendinopathy (CIAT) is a relatively common musculoskeletal entity that results in significant pain and disability. Elias and colleagues[1] studied 40 subjects with a diagnosis of CIAT and found an average preoperative American Orthopaedic Foot and Ankle Society ankle-hindfoot (AOFAS-AH) score of 56.3, with

Disclosures: The authors have no disclosures related to the production of this article.
Division of Foot and Ankle Surgery, West Penn Hospital, Allegheny Health Network, 4800 Friendship Avenue, Pittsburgh, PA 15224, USA
* Corresponding author.
E-mail address: acatanzariti@faiwp.com

Clin Podiatr Med Surg 33 (2016) 113–123
http://dx.doi.org/10.1016/j.cpm.2015.07.002
0891-8422/16/$ – see front matter © 2016 Elsevier Inc. All rights reserved.

an average preoperative visual analog scale score of 7.5. In a retrospective study of 29 procedures, Den Hartog[2] found significantly lower functional scores before flexor hallucis longus (FHL) transfer for CIAT, with an average preoperative AOFAS-AH score of 41.7. CIAT often includes retrocalcaneal bursitis, Haglund deformity, insertional calcification, insertional paratenonitis, insertional tendinosis, equinus deformity, and, sometimes, systemic enthesopathies. The pathogenesis of CIAT is unclear. Advanced imaging, especially MRI, can provide prognostic information to guide treatment. Unfortunately, the success rate with nonsurgical treatment decreases significantly once intrasubstance changes consistent with tendinosis are present on MRI.[3] In 24% to 45.5% of patients with Achilles tendinopathy, conservative management is unsuccessful and surgery has to be considered.[4] Surgery should be considered in patients who experience refractory disease, disability, weakness, and MRI changes consistent with tendinosis. Furthermore, it is important to keep in mind that long-standing disease is associated with poor surgical outcomes and a greater rate of reoperation.[5] Therefore, the decision to implement nonoperative care for a specific period of time before proceeding with surgery might adversely affect the surgical outcome. The timing of surgery should be based on objective factors, such as clinical findings and MRI results, as well as the patient's response to nonoperative treatment.

CAUSE

The cause of CIAT is most likely multifactorial, with both intrinsic factors (Haglund deformity, muscle weakness, hindfoot malalignment, and high body mass index) and extrinsic factors (inappropriate footwear, training errors, and generalized overuse that results in excessive load on the Achilles tendon) being implicated.[6] In a comparative laboratory study, it was found that the altered production of collagen, an increase in type II and type III, may be a reason for the histopathologic alterations seen with CIAT.[7] The stress-shielded side of the enthesis shows a tendency to develop cartilage-like and/or atrophic changes from lack of tensile load.[8] In a large retrospective study of competitive and recreational athletes with Achilles tendon problems, Kvist[9] reported that 66% had noninsertional tendinopathy, whereas 23% had either retrocalcaneal bursitis or insertional tendinopathy. Johansson and colleagues[10] identified 36 operations that addressed CIAT out of 1425 total operations performed on the Achilles, demonstrating a 2.5% incidence of CIAT. Elias and colleagues[1] describes insertional Achilles tendinopathy as having a bimodal distribution affecting younger athletic individuals involved in activities requiring forceful push-off or bursts of acceleration; whereas the second and most common distribution was found in older sedentary patients with comorbidities.

NONOPERATIVE MANAGEMENT

Nonoperative management for CIAT includes both traditional and nontraditional treatments. Traditional therapies include nonsteroidal antiinflammatory medications, oral steroids, footgear modifications, and posterior muscle group stretching and eccentric exercises. Nontraditional therapies include ultrasound-guided dextrose or polidocanol sclerosing injections, extracorporeal shock wave therapy, and cryoultrasound.[11]

In a 50-subject cohort with chronic pain, subjects managed with repetitive load-energy shockwave therapy demonstrated more favorable results at 4 months than those managed with a 12-week eccentric loading regimen with regard to Victorian Institute of Sports Assessment-Achilles score, pain rating, pain threshold, and tenderness.[12] Significant improvements in pain scores were found after intratendinous injections of 1 mL of 2% lidocaine and 1 mL of 50% dextrose, providing a low-cost and safe treatment with good long-term evidence in 22 cases of CIAT.[13] Although eccentric loading was the common modality found in a systematic review of management of CIAT, the literature suggests that eccentric exercises may not be as effective in the treatment of insertional Achilles tendinopathy as it is in the treatment of midsubstance Achilles tendinopathy.[14] Kearney and Costa,[15] in a systematic review, demonstrated that there is consensus among investigators that conservative treatments should be tried before operate interventions; however, there is no consensus regarding how long conservative measures should be used before they are considered unsuccessful. When considering physical therapy, there should be an understanding that conventional Achilles tendon stretching exercises can aggravate CIAT. Without specific instructions to the therapist, a patient's symptoms can be magnified with physical therapy.

PREOPERATIVE EVALUATION

Preoperative evaluation should include a thorough history of present illness, focusing on factors that directly affect symptoms, especially in patients such as industrial workers, athletes, and so forth. Comorbidities that directly affect CIAT, such as systemic diseases associated with enthesopathies, should be identified.

Key areas of the physical examination should include inspection for specific foot type. Nonneurologic cavus foot deformity is often associated with CIAT, especially when the deformity predominately involves the hindfoot. Both open and closed kinetic chain evaluations are important when evaluating foot deformity. Structural deformity with concomitant malalignment should be addressed during surgical management of CIAT. Focal areas of tenderness within the insertion of the Achilles tendon, as well as other areas of the retrocalcaneal region, should be noted. Hypertrophy and/or nodularity of the Achilles tendon about its insertion should also be noted because these findings are consistent with tendinopathy. Ankle joint range of motion should be evaluated with the knee both extended and flexed because equinus deformity should be identified. It should be ascertained if the deformity involves only the gastrocnemius or the soleus as well. Surgical management addressing the equinus can then be planned accordingly. It is also important to compare muscle tone and calf girth to the contralateral extremity to ascertain the degree of weakness. Additionally, single and double heel rise can also provide information regarding strength. The inability to perform a single heel rise on the affected extremity is consistent with posterior muscle group weakness. The authors often consider transfer of the FHL tendon in these patients.

Radiographic examination, including weightbearing lateral and axial views, is important. Lateral radiographs can identify an increased calcaneal inclination angle, Haglund deformity, a large retrocalcaneal prominence, and calcification about the insertion of the Achilles tendon. Axial views can demonstrate varus deformity as well as calcifications. Debridement of calcifications, enthesophytes and osseous prominences, as well as structural realignment, will be component parts of surgical management.

MRI is very important for preoperative evaluation. The success rate with nonsurgical treatment decreases significantly when intrasubstance changes consistent with tendinosis are present on MRI. Furthermore, long-standing disease is associated with poor surgical outcomes and a greater rate of reoperation. Nicholson and colleagues[3] found that tendons with greater intrasubstance degeneration, as documented on sagittal MRI, often require operative intervention. Thus, patients demonstrating advanced tendinosis in the absence of acute inflammation are likely to require an operative procedure for resolution of their symptoms.[4] In a prospective study of 57 subjects with CIAT, MRI was found to have a sensitivity and specificity of 95% and 50%, respectively.[16] With respect to outcome prediction, Khan and colleagues[16] found that both clinical baseline scores and MRI severity were associated with outcomes. Therefore, MRI can provide prognostic information guiding treatment at various stages of CIAT. The authors obtain MRI on all patients diagnosed with CIAT as a baseline.

SURGICAL MANAGEMENT

Surgical therapy for CIAT should be comprehensive, addressing all pathologic components (Video 1). Principles of surgical management should include

1. Debridement of hypertrophic and diseased Achilles tendon, bursa, enthesophytes, and paratenon.
2. Decompression of the distal Achilles tendon by resection of the posterior superior calcaneal prominence.
3. Tendon reconstruction, which might include regional tissue rearrangements, tendon transfer, or tendon replacement.
4. Posterior muscle group lengthening.
5. Osteotomy of the calcaneus.

Surgery is performed under general inhalation anesthesia with the patient in a prone position. A bump under the contralateral hip will rotate the foot into a better position, especially in obese patients. The surgical table can be further rotated, if necessary; however, the patient must be adequately secured. The authors prefer a well-padded pneumatic thigh tourniquet.

A gastrocnemius recession is considered when equinus is present. This is performed through a linear incision placed distal to the medial head of the gastrocnemius muscle. A gastrocnemius-soleus recession can also be performed if necessary. This is often an intraoperative decision.

A serpentine incision is made over the posterior aspect of the heel. This incision begins just distal to the midsubstance region of the Achilles tendon and extends to the plantar heel (**Fig. 1**). This incision should be long enough to avoid excessive tension on the wound edges. The serpentine nature of this incision also helps to reduce skin tension. This approach permits access to the distal Achilles tendon for

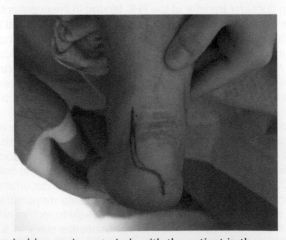

Fig. 1. Serpentine incision made posteriorly with the patient in the prone position.

debridement and repair, ostectomy of the calcaneus, and transfer of the FHL tendon. Care is taken to avoid undermining during dissection. The depth of the proximal portion of this initial incision should extend to the paratenon, whereas the distal portion extends to the periosteum overlying the calcaneus. The paratenon is incised and retracted.

A full-thickness linear incision is then made into the distal Achilles tendon, extending distally onto the calcaneus to the level of bone. All soft tissues are debrided from the posterior calcaneus, including medial and lateral. This allows adequate access to the posterior-superior aspect of the calcaneus. The Achilles tendon has a vast and diffuse insertion into the calcaneus. Enough of the Achilles tendon remains attached to the calcaneus, even after what appears to be extensive dissection, such that the foot will plantarflex with a Thompson test. A sagittal saw is then used to resect a generous portion of bone to adequately decompress the distal aspect of the Achilles tendon (**Fig. 2**). This bone is resected from inferior to superior, with care taken to avoid the subtalar joint. A rasp or burr can be used to smooth any rough areas, especially the medial and lateral borders of the posterior calcaneus.

Further attention is then directed to the medial and lateral segments of the distal Achilles tendon. These portions of the tendon are thoroughly debrided. This should

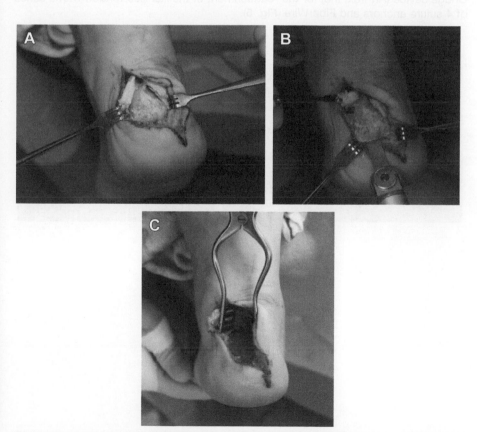

Fig. 2. (A–C) The posterior superior calcaneal prominence is removed using a microsagittal saw.

include any diseased and/or hypertrophic tendon, as well as calcifications within the tendon itself. The tendon will be repaired before closure.

A self–retaining retractor is placed proximally within the incised portion of the Achilles tendon for harvest of the FHL tendon (**Fig. 3**). This provides access to the posterior aspect of the lower leg where the fascia is identified and incised. The FHL muscle belly lies just beneath the fascia. Umbilical tape is placed around the FHL muscle and tendon, which is then traced distally toward the tarsal tunnel. The foot and hallux are maximally plantarflexed, and the FHL tendon is incised just before it enters the tarsal tunnel. The tendon should be cut under complete visualization with care taken to avoid neurovascular injury. The tendon end is then sutured with FiberWire (Arthrex, Inc, Naples, FL, USA) in a whipstitch fashion to prepare for transfer.

The next step is to transfer the FHL tendon into the posterior calcaneus. Various techniques can be used to accomplish transfer. The authors prefer to transfer the tendon as far posterior as possible to maintain the mechanical advantage provided by a long lever arm. Additionally, we prefer to maintain the foot in slight plantar flexion during the transfer. Our preferred technique for FHL tendon transfer is to deliver a biotenodesis screw into the posterior calcaneus (**Fig. 4**).

The Achilles tendon is then reattached to the calcaneus. There are several techniques available to accomplish reattachment. The authors use the Arthrex Speed-Bridge device (Arthrex, Inc) for the reattachment of the Achilles tendon with a series of 4 suture anchors and FiberWire (**Fig. 5**).

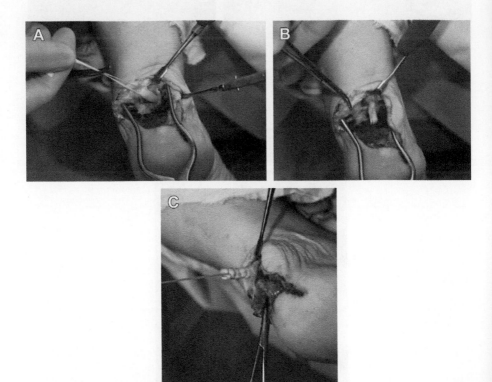

Fig. 3. (*A*) The FHL is identified by splitting the deep fascia anterior to the Achilles. (*B, C*) The FHL is harvested and subsequently sutured to prepare for transfer.

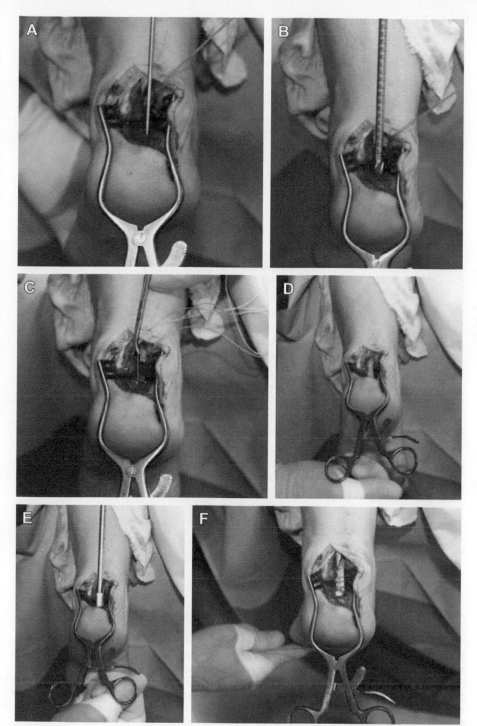

Fig. 4. (*A*) The interference screw guidewire is angled plantar distal through the calcaneus. (*B*) The appropriately sized reamer is drilled over the guide wire creating a transosseous tunnel through the plantar cortex. (*C*) The FiberWire is passed into the tunnel and through the plantar aspect of the heel. (*D*) The tendon is passed into the tunnel and tensioned appropriately with the foot in slight plantarflexion. (*E*) The appropriately sized biotenodesis screw is inserted into the tunnel while maintaining tension. (*F*) Completed transfer with the suture ends cut.

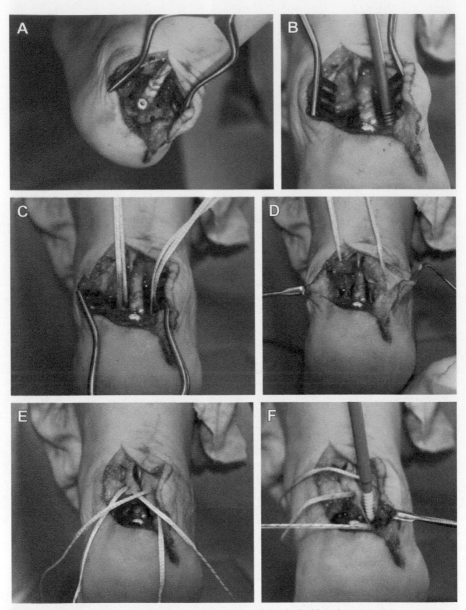

Fig. 5. (*A, B*) Guideholes are drilled and tapped with included hardware in a square pattern avoiding the tendon transfer site. (*C*) Suture anchors are placed in the two proximal holes. (*D*) Suture is passed through the medial and lateral portion of the split Achilles tendon. (*E*) One free suture tail from each anchor is crossed and paired. (*F*) Paired tails are tensioned and inserted into the two distal holes with anchors. (*G*) Completed Achilles SpeedBridge re-attachment and the resultant hourglass configuration of the FiberWire and suture anchors. (*H*) Free tails are cut flush to the distal anchors for a knotless repair and the central portion of the Achilles is then re-approximated with FiberWire.

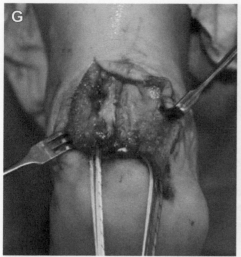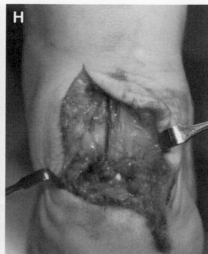

Fig. 5. (*continued*).

The Achilles tendon is then reapproximated side to side with absorbable suture. The paratenon is sometimes closed in a separate layer. Skin closure is then performed in standard fashion.

CALCANEAL OSTEOTOMY

Several studies have investigated open retrocalcaneal decompression and tendon debridement through a variety of approaches. In 1965, Keck and Kelly[17] first described their technique for addressing Haglund deformity. They described 2 types of procedures, the first involved resection of the superior calcaneal prominence and removal of any bursa in the area. The second technique involved removal of a dorsally based wedge from the posterior calcaneus (**Fig. 6**). This can be performed from either a medial or lateral approach. They performed the osteotomy on 5 heels in 4 subjects with 1 good, 2 fair, and 1 poor result. The Keck and Kelly[17] procedure is indicated in patients who show a large Fowler-Philip angle, total angle, and calcaneal inclination angle. These are frequently concomitant with a cavus foot structure.[18] The authors consider this osteotomy in younger athletes who fail nonoperative care with a high calcaneal inclination angle, virtually no calcification within the tendon, and absence of intrasubstance changes on MRI.

POSTOPERATIVE MANAGEMENT

A nonweightbearing short-leg cast or fracture brace is maintained for 3 to 4 weeks. The authors prefer a cast with dorsiflexor pressure on the foot to maintain muscle tension and to reduce the incidence of atrophy during convalescence. Sutures are maintained for approximately 3 weeks. Four-point crutch gait begins in a fracture brace following cast removal and progresses to full weightbearing over the next 2 weeks. Patients are then transitioned from a fracture brace to a supportive shoe at approximately 6 weeks postsurgery. The authors institute physical therapy after patients are ambulating in standard footgear.

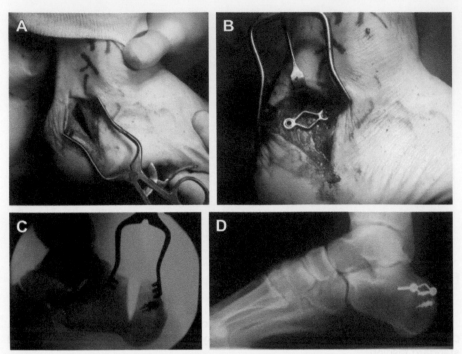

Fig. 6. (A–D) Dorsally based wedge osteotomy at the posterior calcaneus fixated with a claw plate.

SUPPLEMENTARY DATA

Supplementary data related to this article can be found online at http://dx.doi.org/10.1016/j.cpm.2015.07.002.

REFERENCES

1. Elias I, Raikin SM, Besser MP, et al. Outcomes of chronic insertional Achilles tendinosis using FHL autograft through single incision. Foot Ankle Int 2009;30(3): 197–204.
2. Den Hartog BD. Flexor hallucis longus transfer for chronic Achilles tendinosis. Foot Ankle Int 2003;24:233–7.
3. Nicholson CW, Berlet GC, Lee TH. Prediction of the success of non-operative treatment of insertional Achilles tendinosis based on MRI. Foot Ankle Int 2007; 28:472–7.
4. Maffulli N, Sharma P, Luscombe KL. Achilles tendinopathy: aetiology and management. J R Soc Med 2004;97(10):472–6.
5. Maffulli N, Binfield PM, Moore D, et al. Surgical decompression of chronic central core lesions of the Achilles tendon. Am J Sports Med 1999;27:747–52.
6. Johnson KW, Zalavaras C, Thordardson DB. Surgical management of insertional calcific achilles tendinosis with a central tendon splitting approach. Foot Ankle Int 2006;27(4):245–50.
7. Maffulli N, Reaper J, Ewen SW, et al. Chondral metaplasia in calcific insertional tendinopathy of the Achilles tendon. Clin J Sport Med 2006;16(4):329–34.

8. Vogel KG, Ordog A, Pogany G, et al. Proteoglycans in the compressed region of the human tibialis posterior tendon and in ligaments. J Orthop Res 1993;11:68–77.
9. Kvist M. Achilles tendon injuries in athletes. Ann Chir Gynaecol 1991;80:188–201.
10. Johansson KK, Sarimo JJ, Lempainen LL, et al. Calcific spurs at the insertion of the Achilles tendon: a clinical and histological study. Muscles Ligaments Tendons J 2012;2(4):273–7.
11. Roche AJ, Calder JD. Achilles tendinopathy: a review of the current concepts of treatment. Bone Joint J 2013;95-B:1299–307.
12. Rompe JD, Furia J, Maffulli N. Eccentric loading compared with shock wave treatment for chronic insertional achilles tendinopathy: a randomized, controlled trial. J Bone Joint Surg Am 2008;90(1):52–61.
13. Ryan M, Wong A, Taunton J. Favorable outcomes after sonographically guided intratendinous injection of hyperosmolar dextrose for chronic insertional and mid-portion achilles tendinosis. Am J Roentgenol 2010;194:1047–53.
14. Alfredson H, Pietila T, Jonsson P, et al. Heavy-load eccentric calf muscle training for the treatment of chronic Achilles tendinosis. Am J Sports Med 1998;26:360–6.
15. Kearney R, Costa ML. Insertional achilles tendinopathy management: a systematic review. Foot Ankle Int 2010;31:689–94.
16. Khan KM, Forster BB, Robinson J, et al. Are ultrasound and magnetic resonance imaging of value in assessment of Achilles tendon disorders? A two year prospective study. Br J Sports Med 2003;37:149–53.
17. Keck SW, Kelly PJ. Bursitis of the posterior part of the heel: evaluation of surgical treatment of eighteen patients. J Bone Joint Surg Am 1965;47:267–73.
18. Boffeli TJ, Peterson MC. The Keck and Kelly wedge calcaneal osteotomy for Haglund's deformity: a technique for reproducible results. J Foot Ankle Surg 2012;51(3):398–401.

Combined Tendon and Bone Allograft Transplantation for Chronic Achilles Tendon Ruptures

Alan R. Catanzariti, DPM[a],*, Matthew Hentges, DPM[b]

KEYWORDS

- Achilles tendinopathy • Bone-tendon allograft transplantation
- Calcific insertional Achilles tendonitis • Flexor hallucis longus tendon transfer

KEY POINTS

- Achilles tendinopathy involving the distal segment is a disabling condition.
- Surgical management often requires tendon transfer and regional tissue rearrangement.
- This article proposes a bone-tendon allograft transplantation and flexor hallucis longus transfer to address long-segment tendinopathy involving the insertion.

INTRODUCTION

Achilles tendinopathy can result from a chronic degenerative process, such as calcific insertional Achilles tendinitis (CIAT), unrecognized or delayed rupture of the Achilles tendon, or failed Achilles tendon surgery. Tendinopathy involving the Achilles tendon can be a challenging problem, especially when it involves the distal segment inserting into the calcaneus. When tendon degeneration is pronounced and extensive, involving a large segment of the distal Achilles tendon, surgical options are limited. This problem is especially difficult to manage in patients with high-demand occupational requirements who often present with significant disability.

Reconstructive strategies are often limited due to the significant amount of degenerative tendon, both proximal and distal, and the resultant deficit. Traditional techniques such as V-Y advancement flaps,[1] turndown flaps,[2,3] and other synthetic augmentation procedures to repair these large defects have been recommended. The use of Achilles tendon allograft has shown good results in the reconstruction of

a Residency Training Program, Foot & Ankle Surgery, West Penn Hospital, 4800 Friendship Avenue, N1, Pittsburgh, PA 15224, USA; b Foot & Ankle Surgery, West Penn Hospital, 4800 Friendship Avenue, N1, Pittsburgh, PA 15224, USA
* Corresponding author.
E-mail address: acatanzariti@faiwp.com

Clin Podiatr Med Surg 33 (2016) 125–137
http://dx.doi.org/10.1016/j.cpm.2015.07.003
0891-8422/16/$ – see front matter © 2016 Elsevier Inc. All rights reserved.

anterior cruciate ligament tears, patellar tendon ruptures, and biceps tendon ruptures.[4–7] However, its use in the reconstruction of chronic disease of the Achilles tendon is not well reported. Haraguchi and colleagues[4] presented their technique for allograft reconstruction of the Achilles tendon. Their reasons for using this technique include (1) morbidity associated with autogenous tendon transfer is avoided, (2) the amount of autogenous tendon may be insufficient, (3) using allograft reduces overall operating time, and (4) the mechanical properties of Achilles tendon allograft have been demonstrated to be excellent.[4–6] A recent technique article by Hanna and colleagues[8] also demonstrated good results with the use of Achilles tendon allograft.

HISTORY

These patients often present with a chief complaint of disability. Although they have complaints of pain, their inability to function or perform at a certain level is often their primary concern. Disability from work, inability to exercise, generalized difficulty walking, and compensatory gait disturbances with secondary pain are common complaints. Many of these patients describe a slow, insidious process that has developed over several years. Ultimately, this adversely affects their ability to function. Some patients may have experienced an acute rupture of the Achilles tendon for which the diagnosis was delayed or missed. This group of patients may have failed nonoperative therapy and continue to experience persistent pain and disability. The authors have also encountered long-segment distal tendinosis in patients with failed surgery for CIAT. These patients continue to have symptoms following their index procedure, as well as disability that was often absent before surgery. Additionally, some patients can sustain a rupture of the repaired Achilles tendon from its insertion.

Although nonoperative therapy, particularly rest and immobilization, is effective for pain management, these patients have persistent disability. Unfortunately, nonoperative therapy, including aggressive rehabilitation, is often not effective in returning this group of patients back to function.

A medical history demonstrating conditions that might adversely affect healing should be noted and addressed, if possible. Issues include wound healing in poorly controlled diabetes mellitus (hemoglobin A1c >8.0), tobacco use, long-term steroid use, prior Achilles surgery, and pharmaceuticals that negatively affect healing, especially in the Achilles tendon region.

PHYSICAL EXAMINATION

Examination often demonstrates tenderness with palpation of the distal Achilles tendon. The tendon may appear hypertrophic, bulbous, and nodular throughout the distal segment. In cases involving a missed diagnosis of Achilles tendon rupture or rupture of the Achilles tendon from its insertion following surgery for CIAT, the tendon might be absent or very difficult to identify. All patients have weakened plantar flexor power relative to the contralateral extremity. A calf-squeeze test (Thompson test) performed with the patient in a prone position may demonstrate decreased plantar flexion when compared with the contralateral foot. Additionally, when the patient actively flexes the knee in the prone position, the ipsilateral foot may have less plantar flexion.

The ipsilateral calf muscle usually demonstrates a smaller girth and decreased muscle tone in static stance. Patients are often unable to perform a single heel-rise. They have gait disturbances that are typical for a weakened posterior muscle group; some may even demonstrate a calcaneus gait.

IMAGING

Standard lateral and axial radiographs may demonstrate calcification around the insertion of the Achilles tendon into the calcaneus. Although advanced imaging is not critical to diagnosis, MRI can provide information regarding the extent of tendon degeneration. Additionally, MRI can identify tendon degeneration involving the insertion. This information is helpful for surgical planning. Ultrasonography can provide a dynamic assessment of tendon function and also help determine the extent of tendinosis.

RATIONALE FOR TRANSPLANTATION BONE-TENDON ALLOGRAFT

The authors prefer transplantation of a bone-tendon allograft in combination with a flexor hallucis longus (FHL) tendon transfer through an extensile approach to manage long-segment tendinosis involving the distal portion of the Achilles tendon. Advantages of this technique include

1. All diseased tissue is exposed. This often eliminates the source of pain and provides space to accommodate the transplanted allograft.
2. There is no disturbance of the regional anatomy, such as seen with local tissue rearrangements (eg, V-Y advancements, flap-down techniques).
3. Secure attachment of bone-on-bone with compression screws allows adequate incorporation at the host-graft interface. Open kinetic chain exercises can then begin relatively soon following surgery.
4. Space for sufficient volume of allograft as needed is provided.

SURGICAL TECHNIQUE

This procedure is performed with the patient fully secured in a prone position. The authors typically bump the contralateral hip and use a well-padded pneumatic thigh tourniquet. We sometimes prep and drape the contralateral extremity to serve as a guide when tensioning the FHL transfer as well as the transplanted allograft. A full-thickness incision is then made along the posterior aspect of the lower leg extending distally to the plantar skin of the heel (**Fig. 1**). If possible, incisions from previous surgeries should be incorporated. Full-thickness flaps should be developed to the level of the paratenon or tendon. The authors often include the paratenon in the full-thickness flaps if significant scar is present from previous surgeries. Soft tissue undermining should be avoided and we recommend double-prong skin hooks if skin retraction is necessary. This incision should be rather long to minimize tension and all retraction should be deep, avoiding retractors on the skin edges (**Fig. 2**).

The Achilles tendon should then be mobilized and inspected. The diseased segment of tendon should be completely evacuated so that relatively healthy tissue, capable of tenodesis, is present within the remaining stump. Debridement should include all tissue extending to the level of the calcaneus. Any surrounding scar tissue from previous surgery should also be removed (**Figs. 3** and **4**). Adequate space should be developed to accommodate the necessary volume of allograft and to minimize tension on the wound.

The FHL tendon is then harvested in standard fashion through an incision made in the posterior fascia (**Fig. 5**). The FHL muscle belly lies just beneath the fascia. Umbilical tape is placed around the FHL muscle and tendon, which is then traced distally toward the tarsal tunnel (**Fig. 6**). The foot and hallux are maximally plantarflexed, and the FHL tendon is incised just before it enters the tarsal tunnel. The tendon should be cut under complete visualization with care taken to avoid neurovascular injury. The

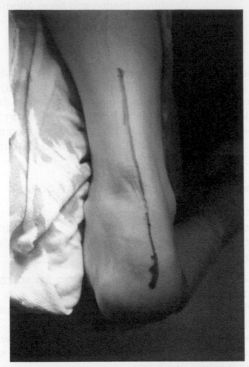

Fig. 1. Extensile incision permitting access to the disease tendon and posterior calcaneus.

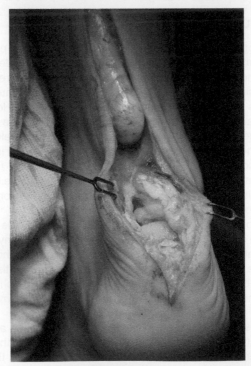

Fig. 2. Degenerated stump of Achilles tendon 6 months status after repair of calcific insertional Achilles tendonitis with subsequent tendon rupture. Double-pronged skin hooks are used for retraction.

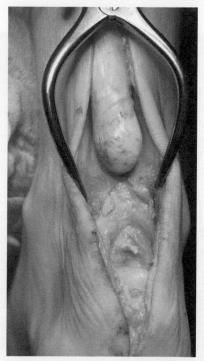

Fig. 3. Substantial degeneration of proximal Achilles stump.

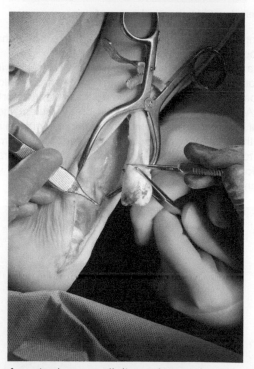

Fig. 4. Debridement of proximal stump. All diseased tissue should be removed to promote side-to-side anastomosis to the allograft tendon.

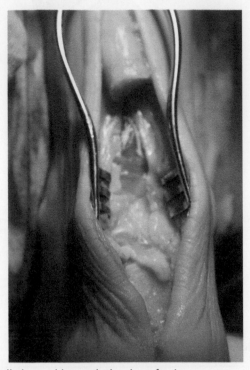

Fig. 5. FHL muscle belly located beneath the deep fascia.

authors do not complete the tendon transfer until after a trough has been created in the calcaneus to accept the bone portion of the allograft.

The allograft bone is then evaluated, especially the depth and width (**Figs. 7** and **8**). A corresponding trough is then developed within the posterior calcaneus. The size of the trough should be sufficient to accommodate a substantial portion of allograft the so that most of the Achilles tendon attachment is preserved and included in the transplantation. However, care must be taken to avoid thinning out the medial, lateral, and plantar borders of the posterior calcaneus. We typically use a small sagittal saw as well as small osteotomes to develop the trough. The medial, lateral, and plantar portions of the posterior calcaneus should be maintained and care should be taken to avoid stress risers in these areas (**Figs. 9** and **10**).

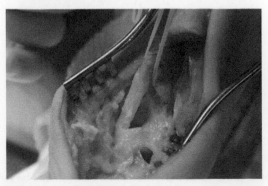

Fig. 6. FHL tendon is isolated and prepared for harvest.

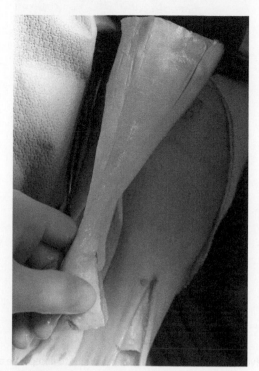

Fig. 7. Achilles tendon allograft and attached calcaneal bone block.

The FHL tendon is then transferred into the dorsal aspect of the trough. Using this dorsal site leaves room for compression screws to secure the allograft bone block to the calcaneus. This is typically performed with an interference screw technique. The tendon is placed under adequate tension with the foot in a plantarflexed position and a biotenodesis screw is delivered to secure the transfer. The authors often assess the contralateral foot when trying to ascertain the appropriate tension for an FHL tendon transfer.

The bone allograft is then remodeled to fit snugly into the trough (**Figs. 11** and **12**). The outer portion of the allograft should not protrude or be proud. This is then pounded

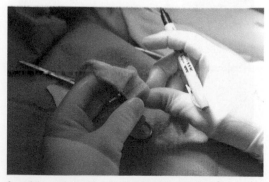

Fig. 8. Evaluation of width and depth of calcaneal bone block.

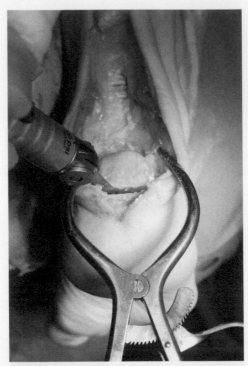

Fig. 9. A trough is developed within the posterior calcaneus to accept the allograft bone block.

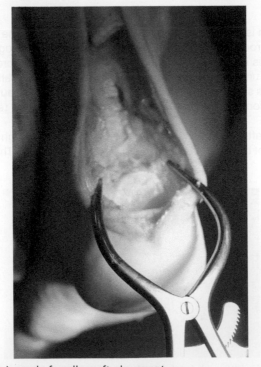

Fig. 10. The trough is ready for allograft placement.

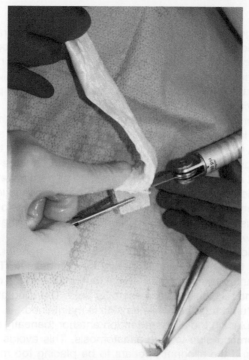

Fig. 11. The calcaneal bone block is remodeled to fit securely into the calcaneal trough.

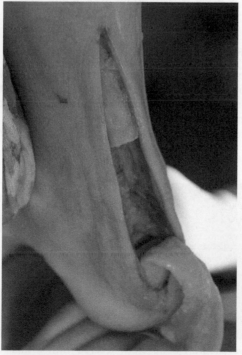

Fig. 12. Allograft bone block with Achilles tendon placed into trough.

in place with a large-surface area tamper with care to avoid fracture. Two small-diameter compression screws are then delivered to secure the allograft bone in place. We suggest countersinking the screws to avoid screw head prominence that might cause heel counterirritation from shoes. Screws should be delivered under image intensification, engaging the plantar calcaneal cortex, which provides adequate compression that will secure the allograft (**Fig. 13**).

The tendon portion of the allograft is then remodeled based on the size of the defect (**Figs. 14** and **15**). A large-diameter nonabsorbable suture used in a Kessler or Bunnell technique is placed within the allograft tendon. This is then used to provide proximal tension on the allograft. A similar type of technique with a large-diameter suture is placed into the host Achilles stump. It will be used to provide distal tension when performing a side-to-side anastomosis. Or the suture can be continued into the allograft tendon for end-to-end anastomosis. In most cases, the authors prefer a side-to-side anastomosis because residual tendinosis is often present in the remaining Achilles tendon stump following debridement.

Tension of the allograft is built around the FHL tendon transfer. However, we also evaluate tension in the contralateral extremity for comparison. The goal is to have somewhat more plantar flexion on the surgical foot relative to the other limb, knowing that muscle tone and tension will decrease over time. The allograft and host Achilles tendon are then sutured together while tension is maintained.

We recommend placing the allograft tendon anterior (beneath) to the host Achilles tendon when performing side-to-side anastomosis. This avoids excess tension on the wound margins. If the allograft appears to be placing too much tension on the skin before closure, the allograft can be sutured to the underlying FHL muscle belly to make it less prominent (**Fig. 16**). Closure is then performed in layers. Closure must be meticulous to avoid tension on the wound and excess handling of the skin margins.

POSTOPERATIVE CARE

The foot should be plantarflexed to avoid skin tension; however, we prefer some dorsiflexion pressure to maintain muscle tone during the nonweightbearing period. We avoid gravity-dependent casts due to potential muscle atrophy of the FHL. Patients should be kept nonweightbearing for approximately 6 weeks. Serial radiographs should be obtained to evaluate incorporation at the host-graft interface. Patients begin

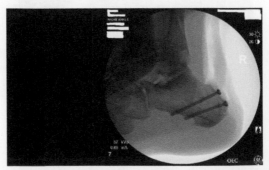

Fig. 13. Intraoperative allograft bone block secured with 2 small-diameter screws. The screws should engage the plantar cortex to enhance compression.

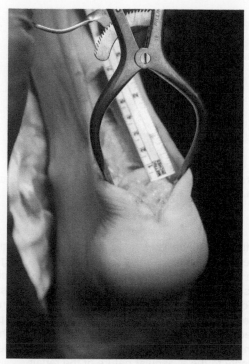

Fig. 14. The defect remaining following debridement is being measured.

partial weightbearing in a fracture brace and progress to full weight as tolerated. They are transitioned into a sneaker and begin a course of rehabilitation.

DISCUSSION

The authors have been using this technique since the mid-2000s and have found this technique especially advantageous for cases of chronic insertional Achilles tendinosis involving a substantial portion of the distal segment. In these patients, there is diffuse

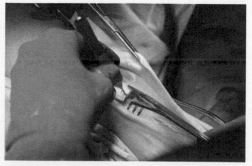

Fig. 15. Tendon portion of allograft is being remodeled to fill the defect.

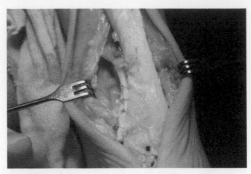

Fig. 16. The allograft tendon is sutured to the underlying FHL muscle and tendon to decrease skin tension.

disease at the insertion of the Achilles tendon. Following debridement of the diseased portion of the Achilles tendon, the resultant gap is often rather large (**Figs. 17** and **18**). In this instance, the Achilles bone-tendon allograft allows for secure fixation of both distal and proximal segments. The use of internal fixation helps to stabilize the allograft bone for incorporation into host bone. A modified Krackow or Bunnell suture construct is used to secure the allograft to the proximal native tendon under physiologic tension. All of our patients received an FHL tendon transfer. We perform this for 2 reasons: (1) to increase the strength of the overall repair and (2) the FHL muscle belly might help to increase the vascularity to the avascular nature of the repair.

We have not observed any evidence of immunologic rejection of the allograft or transmission of disease to the host. Screening of donors is an important component of allograft procurement and all biological tissue carries some risk of bacterial, viral, or prior disease transmission.[9] The American Association of Tissue Banks is responsible for establishing the standards for donor screening as well as serologic and microbiologic testing. Current standards include testing for human immunodeficiency virus, hepatitis B and C infection, hepatitis C virus, and syphilis. The estimated risk of transmission of viral disease from an adequately screened donor is approximately 1 in 1,500,000.[9] Other possible complications include wound necrosis, infection, rerupture, and sural nerve injury.

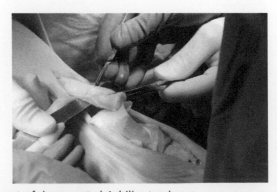

Fig. 17. Debridement of degenerated Achilles tendon.

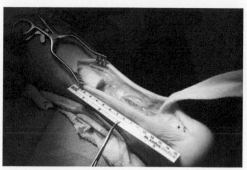

Fig. 18. Remaining deficit following debridement can be rather substantial.

REFERENCES

1. Linn RM, Fischer DA, Smith JP, et al. Achilles tendon allograft reconstruction of the anterior cruciate ligament-deficient knee. Am J Sports Med 1993;21:825–31.
2. McNally PD, Marcelli EA. Achilles allograft reconstruction of a chronic patellar tendon rupture. Arthroscopy 1998;14:340–4.
3. Sanchez-Sotelo J, Morrey BF, Adams RA, et al. Reconstruction of chronic ruptures of the distal biceps tendon with use of an achilles tendon allograft. J Bone Joint Surg Am 2002;84:999–1005.
4. Haraguchi N, Bluman EM, Myerson MS. Reconstruction of chronic Achilles tendon disorders with Achilles tendon allograft. Tech Foot Ankle Surg 2005;4:154–9.
5. Nellas ZJ, Loder BG, Wertheimer SJ. Reconstruction of an Achilles tendon defect utilizing an Achilles tendon allograft. J Foot Ankle Surg 1996;35:144–8.
6. Lepow GM, Green JB. Reconstruction of a neglected achilles tendon rupture with an achilles tendon allograft: A case report. J Foot Ankle Surg 2006;45:351–5.
7. Cienfuegos A, Holgado MI, Diaz del Rio JM, et al. Chronic Achilles rupture reconstructed with Achilles tendon allograft. a case report. J Foot Ankle Surg 2013;52:95–8.
8. Hanna T, Dripchak P, Childress T. Chronic achilles rupture repair by allograft with bone block fixation: technique tip. Foot Ankle Int 2014;35(2):168–74.
9. Robertson A, Nutton RW, Keating JF. Current trends in the use of tendon allografts in orthopaedic surgery. J Bone Joint Surg Br 2006;88(8):988–92.

Surgical Correction of Rigid Equinovarus Contracture Utilizing Extensive Soft Tissue Release

Christopher L. Reeves, DPM, MS, FACFAS[a,b,*],
Amber M. Shane, DPM, FACFAS[b,c],
Francesca Zappasodi, DPM[d], Trevor Payne, DPM[d]

KEYWORDS

- Cavus foot • Cavovarus foot • Spastic equinovarus • Contracture
- Ischemic contracture • Soft tissue release • Tenotomy

KEY POINTS

- A rigid equinovarus contracture of the foot can develop after a cerebrovascular accident, traumatic brain injury, or ischemic event.
- The muscular balance of the lower limb is disrupted secondary to upper motor neuron insult, resulting in a plantarflexed and inverted foot from overactivity of the gastrosoleal complex, tibialis posterior, and the deep flexors.
- Equinovarus contracture patients often are nonambulatory and suffer from pain and traumatic falls as a result of a nonfunctional foot and are predisposed to fractures and ulcerations.
- Release of the Achilles, flexor tendons, peroneal tendons, and the plantar fascia in conjunction with a pie-crusting skin technique can be an effective and minimally invasive way to produce a plantigrade foot that can be successfully braced and functional for transferring and community ambulation.

Financial Disclosure: The authors have nothing to disclose as it relates to the content of this article.
Conflict of Interest: Nothing to report.
[a] Orlando Foot and Ankle Clinic, 2111 Glenwood Drive, Suite 104, Winter Park, FL 32792, USA;
[b] Department of Podiatric Surgery, Florida Hospital East Orlando Surgical Residency Program, 7727 Lake Underhill Road, Orlando, FL 32828, USA; [c] Orlando Foot and Ankle Clinic, 250 North Alafaya Trail, Suite 115, Orlando, FL, USA; [d] Florida Hospital East Orlando Residency Training Program, 7727 Lake Underhill Road, Orlando, FL 32828, USA
* Corresponding author. Orlando Foot and Ankle Clinic, 2111 Glenwood Drive, Suite 104, Winter Park, FL 32792.
E-mail address: docreeves1@yahoo.com

Clin Podiatr Med Surg 33 (2016) 139–152
http://dx.doi.org/10.1016/j.cpm.2015.06.009
0891-8422/16/$ – see front matter © 2016 Elsevier Inc. All rights reserved.

podiatric.theclinics.com

INTRODUCTION

Although deforming contractures of the lower extremities after acute cerebrovascular events are well documented in the literature, there is limited literature regarding specific surgical considerations for the correction of these deformities, which are nonosseus in nature. The equinovarus foot, regardless of its origin, is a challenging pathologic condition for the foot and ankle surgeon. It is critical to have a firm understanding of the cause and symptoms behind an equinovarus deformity before treatment can be implemented. Patients that have suffered acute cerebral or peripheral vascular insults often result in lower extremity contractures that can progress to a rigid state with time. These deformities are often not amenable to bracing and result in high risks of instability and falls in conjunction with the development of pressure lesions. In addition, these patients are generally a fragile population that faces increased risks of morbidity as a result of their sedentary lifestyle and global muscle weakness and are not good candidates for definitive procedures such as a pantalar arthrodesis. The ultimate goal for these patients is to produce a plantigrade foot that can be braced for transfer and ambulation related to daily-living activities. In this article, the clinical presentation of these affected individuals is discussed with special attention to deformities in adults with rigid equinovarus deformities after cerebrovascular-related accidents or peripheral ischemic events. In addition, the subsequent treatment that has been implemented by means of extensive soft tissue releases to construct a balanced and plantigrade foot that is conducive for bracing and fulfills the functional requirements for transferring is discussed.

CAUSE

The upper motor neuron damage caused in cerebrovascular accidents (CVAs) and traumatic brain injuries (TBI) can produce musculoskeletal deformities in addition to cognitive defects.[1] Initially, after these injuries, patients experience hypotonia, hyporeflexia, and flaccid paralysis. Over time, the upper motor neuron disruption seen in these injuries results in increased muscle tone in certain muscle groups and causes an imbalance of the lower extremity muscles, leading to lower extremity spastic deformities. An equinovarus foot deformity is the most common deformity to occur after a CVA. This foot deformity may be spastic in nature or progress to a rigid contracture over time. In addition, acute limb ischemia from a peripheral vascular occlusion can similarly result in these musculoskeletal contractures. Patients with a resultant equinovarus deformity after experiencing a CVA or peripheral ischemic event could be at a considerably higher risk for developing complicated wounds and requiring limb amputation.[2] Before treating these complex deformities, it is essential to obtain a thorough history and physical examination while appreciating the anatomy and biomechanics behind an equinovarus deformity. Treatment of these severe deformities should be individualized and can benefit from aggressive soft tissue releases with subsequent bracing for long-term preservation of function.

BIOMECHANICS

The gait cycle is reliant on normal antagonistic muscle groups working to drive the vector forces of bones and joints to absorb ambulation pressures and provide rigidity for propulsion. There are several intrinsic and extrinsic muscle pairings that contribute to this overall process. One specific antagonistic muscle pair that acts at the level of the ankle joint is the tibialis anterior and peroneus longus, which dorsiflex and plantarflex the first ray, respectively. The peroneus brevis and posterior tibial muscles are also antagonistic in function. The peroneus brevis is responsible for everting the foot, while the posterior tibial muscle acts to invert the hindfoot. Another important muscle pairing is the antagonistic pull of the triceps surae and the long extensors of the anterior compartment, which plantarflex and dorsiflex the foot and the ankle, respectively. The foot itself has antagonistic muscle groups, the intrinsic and extrinsic extensors and flexors, which work in tandem to keep the toes straight with a counterbalanced pull at the metatarsophalangeal joint and inter-phalangeal joints.[3]

Disruption of these critical muscular balances in the foot after neurologic injury incurred from CVAs or from acute peripheral ischemic events can result in an equino-varus foot deformity that is of limited function.

CLINICAL PRESENTATION

Patients that have suffered CVAs or TBI may present with a spastically contracted foot in an equinovarus position that is of minimal function secondary to neurologic insult. These patients are often nonambulatory and have difficulty transferring because of their foot deformities. Patients with a long-standing spastic equinovarus deformity can progress to a rigid contracted state (**Fig. 1**). This patient population often shows signs of gait instability, frequent falls, and foot pain. In addition, this patient population can develop plantar callosities and pressure ulcerations that can become limb threatening.[4]

CLINICAL EVALUATION

In ambulatory patients, notation of the wear pattern of a patient's shoe can give some early indications as to load-bearing abnormalities and can correlate to osseous prom-inences or areas of increased pressure on the foot.[5] Clawing of the toes, a cocked up hallux, high arches, and plantar prominence of the lateral foot should all be noted on initial visual examination. The integrity of the skin should be examined in detail and any calluses or ulcerations thoroughly evaluated. The patient's vascular status should be

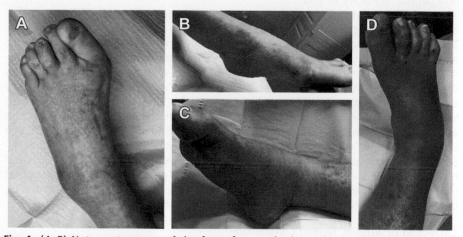

Fig. 1. (A–D) Note contractures of the feet after cerebral vascular accident with the long flexors overpowering the noncontributory anterior muscle group. Visual representation of accentuated plantar flexion with inversion causing increased pressure on the lateral soft tis-sues of the foot translating to significant potential for ulceration and possible limb loss.

assessed carefully, particularly in patients that have suffered a CVA and therefore have a predilection for vascular disease.[2] Range of motion of the ankle, rearfoot, midfoot, and forefoot joints can offer details about the degree of rigidity of the foot and should be examined judiciously and compared with the contralateral lower extremity. The muscle strength of opposing muscle groups of the lower extremity should be graded to identify weaknesses or hyperactivity. Testing of the Achilles and patellar reflexes can also be revealing in patients who have upper motor neuron injury. These patients may have hyperreflexia as well as signs of clonus, positive Babinski sign, and muscle spasticity. The gastrosoleal complex should be examined using the Silfverskiold test, which can be helpful with operative planning of a tendo Achilles lengthening versus gastrocnemius recession. It is of note that this test is only reliable in patients with a static, nonspastic, and equinovarus deformity and should not be used to evaluate patients with a spastic equinovarus deformity.[1]

The clinical examination should also include a standing and gait evaluation if the patient is able. Often, post-CVA patients are nonambulatory and may have difficulty standing for this portion of the examination. When possible, the practitioner should evaluate the relationship of the long axis of the tibia to the calcaneus while facing the standing patient from behind.

SURGICAL TECHNIQUES
Preoperative Considerations

Surgical intervention should be considered after conservative therapies such as bracing and physical therapy have been exhausted or are impractical for the patient because of the level of deformity. Preoperatively, it should be recognized that many of these patients have poor nutrition status and sedentary lifestyles that are associated with decreased healing rates. These patients are not good candidates for high-demand surgeries such as arthrodesis procedures, which place them in long-term rehabilitation facilities and place a great amount of physical stress on the patient. Correction of these deformities with external fixation is also associated with risks in these patients. There are increased risks of falls because of the cumbersome hardware and pin site morbidity as well.

An extensive review of the literature regarding specific surgical intervention with strictly soft tissue procedures, in these patients with rigid deformities, was sparse. To the authors' knowledge, this is the only review that details multiple options for soft tissue release and augmentations with tendon transfers for the purpose of correcting a rigidly contracted equinovarus foot. After a CVA, it can take patients 6 to 9 months for neurologic recovery after such an insult. Because of this timeline, surgery should not be performed earlier than 6 months after a CVA when spontaneous neurologic recovery can occur.[2] Soft tissue releases in adult patients with static or spastic acquired equinovarus can play an important role in producing a plantigrade foot. In a spastic contracted equinovarus foot in a post-CVA setting, there is often overactivity of the gastrocnemius-soleus complex and tibialis posterior tendon producing an equinovarus foot. The ultimate goal in these patients is to construct a balanced foot that can be successfully braced and used for daily transfer, while preventing callus and ulcer formation and reducing the risk of falls, pain, and limb loss.

Correction of Achilles Tendon Contracture

A contracted Achilles tendon is often a major driving force in the rigid equinus deformity seen in patients that have experienced a CVA. Complete isolated release of this tendon can be approached through a small stab incision just medial or lateral to the tendon, 3 cm from its insertion on the calcaneus. A number 15 blade should be inserted parallel and just anterior to the tendon and turned perpendicular to the tendon through the incision, releasing the tendon fibers completely, with care taken not to penetrate the overlying skin posteriorly. Once the tenotomy is complete, the ankle should be dorsiflexed and the relationship of the foot and ankle re-evaluated. Release of the Achilles tendon can also be completed through the incision described for release of the flexor hallucis longus, flexor digitorum longus, and tibialis posterior tendons.

Correction of Flexor Hallucis Longus, Flexor Digitorum Longus, and Tibialis Posterior Tendon Contractures with Tarsal Tunnel Decompression

Tenotomies and tendon sectioning of the deep posterior muscle group can be approached through a posterior medial-based incision over the tarsal tunnel. The incision should be made 2.5 cm posterior to the medial malleolus and extended inferiorly to the abductor hallucis muscle belly. The incision should measure 5 to 7 cm in length for adequate visualization of tendinous structures. The incision is made with a number 15 blade through skin and deepened until the flexor retinaculum is identified. At this time, the flexor retinaculum is identified and incised with a number 15 blade, with care taken to protect the underlying neurovascular structures. Next, the tibialis posterior tendon should be identified and isolated from its fibrocartilaginous tunnel and is the most anterior tendon noted in the tarsal tunnel. It is recommended that a tenotomy is performed and a 2-cm section of the tendon be removed, to prevent scarring down and recurrence of equinovarus deformity. The flexor digitorum longus and flexor hallucis longus tendons can then be isolated and systematically released and sectioned until the talocalcaneal relationship is restored. This incision also allows for access to release the Achilles tendon if needed. In addition, with long-standing cavovarus contractures, one would expect to see shortening of the medial soft tissue structures. Acute correction to a rectus foot can place traction on the medial structures and risk neurovascular embarrassment. As a result, it is essential to decompress the contents of the tarsal tunnel during the reconstructive procedures.

Correction of Posterior Capsular Contracture

When release of the Achilles tendon provides insufficient correction of the equinus deformity, release of the posterior ankle and subtalar joint capsules should be performed. This release can be performed through the previously described incision to access the deep flexor tendons or through an open Achilles approach. The transected ends of the Achilles tendon from previous tenotomy are identified and retracted proximally and distally, allowing for exposure of Kager triangle. After blunt dissection through lipomatous tissue, the posterior capsular fibers can be identified. Next, the posterior capsule is sharply incised and released with Littler scissors, with care taken to protect the underlying tendinous and neurovascular structures.

Correction of Peroneus Longus and Peroneus Brevis Tendon Contractures

Release of the peroneus longus and peroneus brevis tendons may also be required to completely reduce an equinovarus contracted foot. Although certainly not as common, the peroneal tendons can contribute to residual equinus deformity and limit a full reduction of the deformity. The approach for release of these tendons is through a laterally based incision made 4 cm proximal to the lateral malleolus and 2 cm posterior to the posterior border of the fibula. The incision is 4 cm in length and made longitudinally with a number 15 blade along the course of the tendons. The incision is deepened through skin and subcutaneous structures until the corresponding tendon sheaths are visible. Once the sheaths are incised, the tendons are isolated and a Z-tendon lengthening can be performed or a tenotomy with resection of a 2-cm portion of tendon can be performed.

Plantar Fascial Release

Plantar fasciotomies, although typically used in the treatment of pediatric or adolescent patients with a pes cavus deformity, play a role in treating an acquired spastic equinovarus deformity in patients that have suffered a CVA.[6] It is not typically an isolated procedure, but instead performed in conjunction with tenotomies and capsular releases to produce a rectus and plantigrade foot. The plantar fasciotomy is approached through the posterior medial incision previously described for tenotomies of the deep flexor tendons. The inferior-most portion of this incision can be lengthened until it reveals the medial band of the plantar fascia and the abductor hallucis muscle belly. The plantar fascia can be isolated superiorly and inferiorly using a freer elevator and subsequently released with Mayo scissors, with careful consideration of the neurovascular bundle. It is recommended that the fascia is sectioned completely and a wedge removed to prevent scarring down and recurrence of plantar contracture.

Skin Plasty with Pie-Crusting Technique

A long-standing rigid equinovarus deformity may lead to an overlying skin contracture that needs to be addressed during surgical correction. The skin over the medial aspect of the foot tightens over time while in the equinovarus position, just like the underlying soft tissues and tendons. When an aggressive release of tendons and soft tissue is performed, the contracted skin may inhibit reduction of the foot and even threaten the viability of the skin, as the increased tension may cause vascular compromise. A simple pie-crusting technique can be implemented to increase the flexibility of the skin to accommodate the reduction. A number 11 blade is inserted perpendicular to the contracted skin and used to create small holes in the epidermal and dermal skin layers of the tensioned area. This technique is analogous to meshing techniques when performing split thickness skin grafting. Incisions should be at least 2 mm apart from one another with care taken not to plunge deeply, because this may cause injury to underlying structures (Fig. 2).

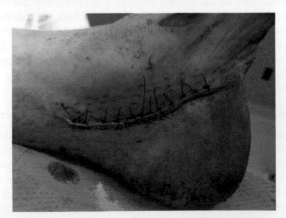

Fig. 2. Pie-crusting skin plasty technique for primary closure over contracted skin areas following extensive soft tissue release.

Complications

When performing release of the flexor tendons, there is a risk to injuring the corresponding neurovascular structures in the area. Careful surgical dissection with blunt instruments can prevent trauma to these vital structures. As with any surgery, there is always a risk of soft tissue infection and wound healing, especially in these particularly fragile post-CVA patients that may have additional comorbidities. The possibility of recurrence of deformity should be low if adequate sections of tendon and ligament are removed during the soft tissue release and patient is braced early in the postoperative process to maintain reduction of the foot.

Case Report 1

A 57-year-old diabetic man presented to our office after suffering a 100% embolic occlusion of his right femoral artery, secondary to an acute thrombus. The patient had vascular intervention in the form of a thrombectomy and femoral-posterior tibial artery bypass to restore vascular perfusion to the ischemic extremity. In addition, the patient underwent fasciotomies of the anterior, lateral, superficial, and deep posterior compartments of the right leg. Following emergent intervention, the limb was salvaged; however, the patient subsequently developed a lower leg contracture (**Fig. 3**). The contracture progressed to a rigid, equinovarus deformity, which resulted in multiple wounds on the lateral aspect of the right foot and eventually led to the development of chronic pain and depression in the patient. Multiple conservative and surgical therapies were instituted over a period of 4 months for this patient and included hyperbaric

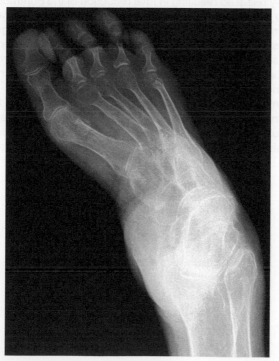

Fig. 3. Preoperative anteroposterior (AP) radiograph of equinovarus contracture after acute peripheral ischemic injury.

oxygen therapy, multiple serial debridements of the lower extremity wounds with negative pressure wound therapy, and split thickness skin grafting.

As a result of his acquired and rigid equinovarus contracture, the patient was restricted to a wheelchair while losing the ability to ambulate. After 7 months of physical therapy, there was no reduction of contracture. In addition, the patient was also nonresponsive to bracing because of his high level of deformity, with no improvement his pain in the right leg and foot. After educating the patient on soft tissue reconstruction in contrast to osseous fusion, which would require substantially more recovery time, the patient elected to move forward with soft tissue reconstruction. A team-oriented surgical approach was taken with vascular surgery to correct the deformity with a posterior release and posterior tibial tendon transfer while avoiding damage to the bypass grafts placed during the initial vascular salvage of the leg.

During the surgical intervention, no tourniquet was used in an effort to prevent damage to the previous vascular grafts. Our vascular surgeon colleague used ultrasound to map the right lower extremity arterial system and bypass grafts intraoperatively. After confirmed patency, we decided to address the posterior contracture using a 6-cm curvilinear incision made directly lateral to the Achilles tendon, where a Z-type lengthening of the Achilles was performed to allow reduction of the contracture. Stepwise testing to measure the degree of contracture reduction was performed after each procedure and, at this point, the contracture was improved but still present. Next, we addressed the contracted flexor tendons through a medial-based incision on the foot over the tarsal tunnel (**Fig. 4**). This release allowed for increased mobility of the foot; however, there were additional soft tissue constrictions around the posterior ankle and subtalar joint capsule. Therefore, the posterior ankle and subtalar joint capsules were sharply released resulting in total reduction of the contracture with the foot positioned 90° to the ground in plantigrade position (**Fig. 5**). To ensure that the progressive deforming force of the posterior tibial tendon did not progress, a posterior tibial tendon transfer through the interosseous membrane was performed. Final intraoperative assessment of the reduced contractures was performed with good anatomic reduction achieved. Layered anatomic closure was completed; a well-padded below-knee cast was applied.

The patient remained non-weight-bearing for 8 weeks and then transitioned to a removable walking boot. Increased edema led to wound dehiscence, which was treated successfully with compression therapy and specialized wound care. A custom ankle-foot orthosis was fitted for the patient; however, the patient chose not to wear it.

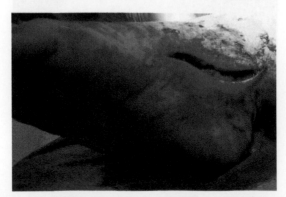

Fig. 4. Intraoperative image showing medially oriented curvilineal incisional approach to flexor tendons, plantar fascial band, and capsular releases.

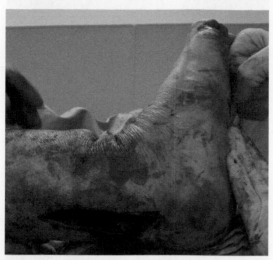

Fig. 5. Intraoperative image demonstrating reduction of equinovarus contracture. Lateral incisional approach shown for release of the posterior capsular structures and Achilles tendon as well as flexors.

Hammertoe contractures developed, which were surgically corrected without complications. Five years postoperatively, the patient is ambulating unassisted without the equinovarus deformity. The patient has continued to experience lymphedema secondarily to the initial ischemic event, and long-term compression therapy has been used (**Fig. 6**).

Case Report 2

An 83-year-old woman presented to the office with a chief complaint of bilateral foot contractures. The patient had a severe reaction to a dopamine antagonist, haloperidol, which caused severe dystonia to both feet and subsequently developed an equinovarus contracture (**Fig. 7**). Before the drug reaction, the patient was able to ambulate independently without difficulty while performing activities of daily living. On presentation to our clinic, she was unable to walk or carry out basic daily functions without direct assistance.

Physical examination of the patient included a comprehensive review of the patient's dermatologic, vascular, neurologic, and musculoskeletal systems. Although the patient was in a contracted equinovarus position, there were no open lesions noted. She did have hyperkeratotic skin lesions present along the maximal point of pressure laterally on the forefoot with reddened, tender skin. Bilaterally, pedal pulses were faint but palpable. Capillary refill time was also delayed to 5 seconds for all digits bilaterally. Her equinovarus deformity was nonreducible with soft tissue contractures of the Achilles tendon and deep flexors. Extensive discussion regarding the risks and benefits of a potential reconstruction took place with the patient and family present. Ultimately, the patient elected to pursue surgical reconstruction of her right foot.

The procedure began with exposure of the posterior aspect of the right leg where rigid contracture of the Achilles tendon was isolated. A transverse tenotomy of the tendon was performed 3 cm proximal to its insertion, after a longitudinal incision was made lateral to the tendon. After the tenotomy was completed, we wanted to

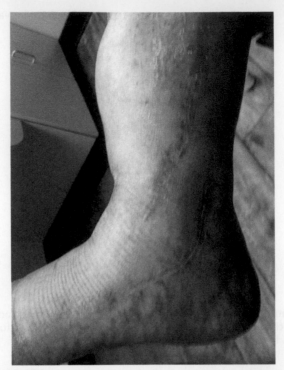

Fig. 6. Eight-week postoperative image with medial incisional well-healed and no residual equinovarus contracture.

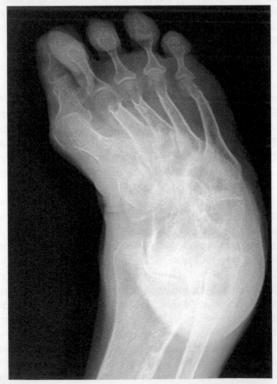

Fig. 7. Preoperative AP radiograph of right foot equinovarus contracture.

ensure that the tendon would not simply readhere, causing a new contracture. There-fore, a 2-cm segment of tendon was resected to prevent relapse of contracture. This procedure alone allowed the foot to reduce to 5° of plantar flexion at the ankle; how-ever, complete reduction of the contracture was not achieved. Next, a second curvi-linear incision was made along the medial aspect of the foot overlying the tarsal tunnel. We commenced our release with the most accessible structures, the flexor retinac-ulum and fascia of the abductor hallucis muscle belly, which were sharply incised. Further dissection was continued along the inferior portion of the incision revealing the plantar fascia, which was sharply transected. Again, to avoid the possibility of contracture recurrence during the healing phase, a 1-cm wedge of the fascia was removed. These soft tissue releases provided increased reduction of the cavovarus deformity with the foot showing significant signs of correction. A stepwise sequential release of the contracted flexor tendons was then performed. The flexor digitorum lon-gus and the flexor hallucis longus tendons were dissected from their tendon sheaths and were transected with a 2-cm segment of tendon removed to prevent reattachment of tendon ends and relapse of contracture. After each tendon was released, the foot was re-evaluated to ascertain the degree of improvement obtained. After reassessing the foot, it had significantly reduced and was nearly perpendicular to the long axis of the tibia. However, there were still noted contractures of the posterior ankle and sub-talar joint capsule preventing the foot from reaching plantigrade position to the ground with some varus contracture still noted as well. Dissection was continued through the existing tarsal tunnel incision until the posterior ankle and subtalar joint capsular fibers were clearly visualized. These structures were then transected in the areas of maximal contracture along the joint lines. At this time, we reassessed the relationship of the foot to the tibia and noted a plantigrade foot, with no residual cavovarus component. In or-der to maintain the stability and reinforce the balance of strength to the new position of the foot, a posterior tibial tendon transfer was performed through a 4-incisional approach. Transposition of the posterior tibial tendon to the central cuboid with a bio-tenodesis screw was completed with tenodesis of the tendon to the extensor tendons with the foot held in maximal dorsiflexion. This tendon transfer ensured stabilization of the foot, and maintenance of the correction was achieved with our aggressive soft tis-sue release (**Fig. 8**). Final intraoperative manipulation of the extremity showed after layered closure, and the patient was placed in a below-knee cast.

The patient's postoperative course was excellent. After 3 weeks in a below-the-knee cast, the patient was progressively encouraged to begin passive range of motion exercises. At 5 weeks after surgery, the patient was progressed to partial weight-bearing for transfer using a walker and CAM boot. Weight-bearing progressed over the next 2 weeks. Finally, the patient was placed in an ankle-foot orthosis 7 weeks af-ter surgery and began a physical therapy regimen with tendon retraining that allowed the patient to graduate to full weight-bearing over a 2-month period. Six months later, the patient underwent correction of the contralateral extremity with maintenance of original correction of right foot (**Fig. 9**). Today, the patient has met her goal and is fully weight-bearing and able to perform her daily activities independently and safely with the use of bilateral ankle and foot orthoses.

Case Report 3

An 86-year-old woman presented to our office after suffering from a severe lower ex-tremity thrombus in the past, which resulted in a progressive cavovarus deformity of the left lower extremity. She also had a previous diagnosis of Parkinson disease. At the initial time of presentation, the patient had extreme difficulty with ambulation

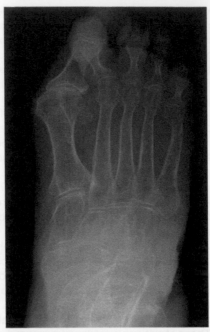

Fig. 8. Postoperative AP radiograph after extensive soft tissue release and posterior tibial tendon transfer.

and required physical assistance. Her goals were to be able to transfer and be ambulatory with the use of a brace for activities of daily living.

On physical examination, there was a noted ulceration on the plantar lateral forefoot. The wound extended to the layer of the deep dermis and had no clinical signs of infection present. Vascular and neurologic examination of the lower extremity was within normal limits. Musculoskeletal evaluation of the left foot revealed a significant equinovarus deformity that was semirigid with no obvious osseous block (**Fig. 10**). Muscle

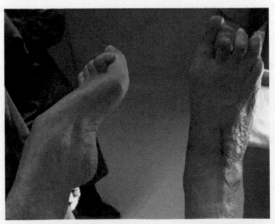

Fig. 9. Comparison of bilateral feet following right foot soft tissue release after 6 months from initial surgery with maintenance of correction.

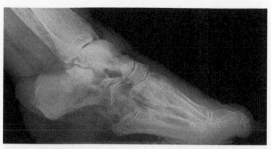

Fig. 10. Preoperative lateral radiograph demonstrating a fixed equinovarus contracture with an incongruous relationship between the tibia and underlying foot.

strength to the anterior muscle group of the left leg was 0/5 and she had limited muscle strength of the remaining muscles of the lower leg due to her underlying neurogenic changes. The foot could not be manually manipulated into a reduced position. There was noted contracture of the gastrosoleal complex, the flexor tendons, and plantar fascia.

The patient's expectations and goals of surgery were discussed extensively, and the patient decided to undergo soft tissue release of the contracted structures. Because of the patient's history of a thrombotic event, hematology was consulted for preoperative recommendations. On being medically cleared, the patient was scheduled for surgery.

The initial focus of the surgery was the equinus component of the foot contracture. A 2-cm linear incision was made just lateral to the Achilles tendon, 3 cm proximal to its insertion. A transverse tenotomy of the tendon was performed, and the foot was maximally dorsiflexed to assess the degree of correction. At this time, the foot was almost perpendicular to the long axis of the tibia. To ensure the maintenance of correction, a 1-cm section of the Achilles tendon was removed at the tenotomy site.

Next, our goal was to address the varus element of the contracture, by exposing the long flexor tendons medially. A curvilinear incision was made along the area of the tarsal tunnel just posterior to the medial malleolus. Blunt dissection was carried down to the flexor retinaculum, which was carefully incised. The neurovascular bundle was cautiously protected while the fascia overlying the muscle belly of the abductor hallucis was also released. Next, a 1-cm segment of the plantar fascia was excised medially through the incision. There was improved positioning of the foot on manual manipulation at this time; however, residual contracture remained that oriented the foot in a varus position. Using the same medial-based incision, the posterior tibial tendon was then identified and transected with a 2-cm section of tendon removed. The flexor digitorum longus and the flexor hallucis longus tendons were also identified in the tarsal tunnel and were noted to be contracted. Both tendons were then transected with a 2-cm portion of each tendon resected. Full correction of the equinovarus deformity was achieved; however, we visually noticed the contracture of the posterior ankle and subtalar joint capsules. The taut capsular fibers were sharply released, and improved mobility was achieved intraoperatively with no additional resistance. Final manipulation of the left foot allowed for complete correction of the equinovarus deformity to a plantigrade foot type (**Fig. 11**).

After anatomic closure of the incisions, the foot was placed in a below-knee cast while held in the corrected position. The patient was kept in a below-knee cast while in a skilled nursing facility with concomitant physical therapy. Within the first 4 weeks, she was able to transfer for daily functions. The patient was then fitted for a pneumatic walking boot and began weight-bearing activities. She gradually increased activity

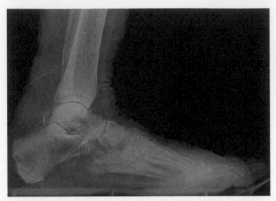

Fig. 11. Lateral radiograph after described soft tissue release. Resolution of equinovarus contracture with plantigrade foot achieved.

and, at 6 weeks postoperatively, she was prescribed an ankle-foot orthosis. Three months from the time of her surgical intervention, the patient was able to ambulate without assistance and complete her daily tasks independently and safely.

SUMMARY

The leading cause of adult spastic foot and ankle deformities is TBI and CVAs. These injuries to the upper motor neurons can lead to a spastic equinovarus deformity of the foot that can progress to a static rigid deformity over time. Often, these patients have pedal callosities or ulcerations and experience difficulty transferring. These patients are excellent candidates for surgical releases of the Achilles tendon, posterior joint capsule, and flexor tendons, when having failed conservative modalities. Treatment should be individualized in each patient, as each presenting deformity can be unique. The overall goals of these soft tissue–based procedures are to reduce pain, reduce risk of ulcerations, and improve quality of life by creating a plantigrade foot that can be successfully braced and functional for transferring.[4]

REFERENCES

1. Keenan M. The management of spastic equinovarus deformity following stroke and head injury. Foot Ankle Clin 2011;16(3):499–514.
2. King B, Ruta D, Irwin T. Spastic foot and ankle deformities: evaluation and treatment. Foot Ankle Clin 2014;19(1):97–111.
3. Marks R. Midfoot and forefoot issues cavovarus foot assessment and treatment issues. Foot Ankle Clin 2008;13:229–41.
4. Boffeli T, Collier R. Minimally invasive soft tissue release of foot and ankle contracture secondary to stroke. J Foot Ankle Surg 2014;53(3):369–75.
5. Rosenbaum AJ, Lisella J. The cavus foot. Med Clin North Am 2014;98:301–12.
6. Weiner D, Jones K, Jonah D, et al. Management of the rigid cavus in children and adolescents. Foot Ankle Clin N Am 2013;18:727–41.

Catastrophic Failure of an Infected Achilles Tendon Rupture Repair Managed with Combined Flexor Hallucis Longus and Peroneus Brevis Tendon Transfer

Devin C. Simonson, DPM[a], Andrew D. Elliott, DPM, JD[b],
Thomas S. Roukis, DPM, PhD[a],*

KEYWORDS

- Complication • Negative pressure wound therapy • Postoperative infection
- Skin graft • Tendon transfer

KEY POINTS

- Significant débridement of infected Achilles tendon rupture repair may preclude primary end-to-end repair.
- Options for repair of such a defect include transfer of the flexor hallucis longus or peroneus brevis tendon or both.
- Combining the transfers of both the flexor hallucis longus and peroneus brevis tendons can adequately restore the power and function of the Achilles tendon.

INTRODUCTION

Achilles tendon (AT) ruptures repaired surgically via an open technique have a high incidence of postoperative wound-healing complications reportedly between 2% and 20%.[1–4] This is often attributed to the location of injury as well as relatively anoxic watershed region of the AT.[1] Of the possible postoperative complications,

---

Financial Disclosure: None reported.
Conflict of Interest: None reported.
[a] Departments of Orthopaedics, Podiatry, and Sports Medicine, Gundersen Health System, 1900 South Avenue, La Crosse, WI 54601, USA; [b] Podiatric Medicine and Surgery Resident (PGY-III), Gundersen Medical Foundation, 1900 South Avenue, La Crosse, WI 54601, USA
* Corresponding author.
E-mail address: tsroukis@gundersenhealth.org

Clin Podiatr Med Surg 33 (2016) 153–162
http://dx.doi.org/10.1016/j.cpm.2015.06.006
0891-8422/16/$ – see front matter © 2016 Elsevier Inc. All rights reserved.

one of the most devastating is a deep infection. When postoperative infection does occur, the area should undergo thorough and systematic débridement and the patient placed on an appropriate course of culture specific antibiotics. As part of the débridement, some or all of the AT may be resected, necessitating delayed reconstruction of the tendon.[1–11] The literature describes numerous techniques for reconstruction, including local tissue advancement, allograft, fascia or tendon autograft, and myotendinous free tissue transfer.[1–4] To maintain ankle joint plantarflexion strength, it is sometimes necessary to transfer surrounding local tendons to supplement the weakened AT or, if the defect is too large, replace it.[1–11] In this case report, the authors present the reconstruction of a chronically infected AT using the flexor hallucis longus (FHL) and peroneus brevis (PB) tendons.

CASE REPORT

The patient is an otherwise healthy 43-year-old man with a past medical history significant for a right AT rupture 12-year prior treated surgically with some plantarflexion weakness and calf atrophy noted. He presented to our Wound Clinic for consultation and ongoing management of a chronic wound following open end-to-end primary repair of his ruptured AT performed 2 months earlier by another provider. During the 2 months before his presentation, the patient experienced ongoing drainage and cellulitis to the surgical site, which had required multiple courses of oral antibiotics and local wound cares.

Our initial physical examination revealed a medially based Achilles incision with persistent dehiscence and intermixed epithelialization. The patient's strength in ankle plantarflexion was decreased and there was an increase in passive dorsiflexion as well. Active range of motion demonstrated 20° of dorsiflexion with minimal effort compared with the contralateral foot, which dorsiflexed 15° with full manual force. There was also an appreciable contour defect and palpable "lump" about the posterior aspect of the lower leg.

Initial débridement in the Wound Clinic did not reveal a sinus tract or deep space abscess however advanced imaging (MRI) was obtained and revealed attenuation of the AT repair with visualized fluid surrounding the suture knots, interstitial edema, and disruption of the tendon fibers. These findings were consistent with failure of the repair and bacterial colonization. Communication between the wound and the repair site was appreciated on MRI (**Fig. 1**). The gastrocnemius and soleus muscles had retracted and the proximal stump of these muscles was enlarged, supporting the belief that the AT repair was compromised and the "lump" on the posterior calf was not the repair but the main proximal tendon stump. Fortunately, his FHL and PB had robust low-lying muscle bellies with no evidence of tendon pathology appreciated. An examination of the distal stump of the AT revealed a sound insertion site. Treatment options included prolonged bracing and intravenous antibiotic use versus a staged surgical débridement with repair of his AT. The patient elected surgical intervention.

SURGICAL TECHNIQUE

Four days after initial presentation, the patient was admitted to our institution for surgical repair of the AT. Although unknown at the time of admission, this would ultimately consist of 3 operations over a 2-week period to successfully débride all diseased and nonviable tissue and transfer both the FHL and PB tendons to the calcaneus. All surgeries were performed by a single surgeon (TSR) under general anesthesia with a

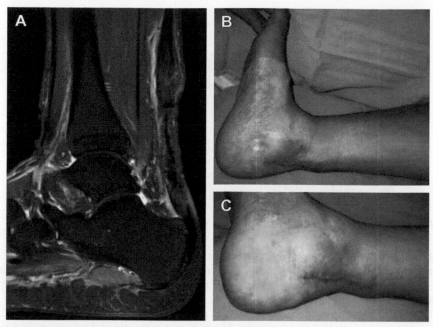

Fig. 1. Preoperative evaluation and clinical photographs. MRI short tau inversion recovery sagittal images demonstrating thickening and heterogeneity of the AT just proximal to the site of prior repair, as well as diffuse subcutaneous edema and enhancement at the lower leg and ankle (*A*). Excessive dorsiflexion noted on physical examination (*B*). Posterior medial nonhealing wound following AT repair (*C*).

single injection popliteal and saphenous block. The patient was placed in the prone position and a thigh tourniquet for hemostasis was used intermittently only as needed.

FIRST SURGERY: DÉBRIDEMENT

Index débridement and wound management followed a standardized protocol used by the senior author (TSR).[12] The original incision was excised and lengthened for adequate exposure. The wound extended directly to the underlying conglomerate of previously placed suture mass and diseased tendon. The AT was noted to be flaccid and without appropriate tension, confirming clinical examination and advanced imaging findings. The tendon itself was severely adhered to the surrounding tissues. Retained sutures were imbedded in the AT and were too numerous to remove (**Fig. 2**). The AT was diseased beyond what would be expected for 6 weeks or more status-post repair. Given these findings, it was deemed most appropriate to resect the AT and suture mass to clean proximal and distal margins. To accomplish this, a 10-cm segment of tendon was resected (**Fig. 3**). The remaining tissues appeared healthy and the skin edges viable. Multiple sets of deep cultures (aerobic, anaerobic, and fungal) were obtained and sent for Gram stain, culture, and sensitivity. The resected AT with retained sutures was sent for pathologic evaluation. The remaining defect was then irrigated via pulsed lavage with a total of 6 L of sterile saline impregnated with 50,000 IU bacitracin (X-Gen Pharmaceuticals, Northport, NY) in each 3-L bag. Antibiotic- impregnated polymethylmethacrylate (PMMA) beads made with 2.4 g of tobramycin (X-Gen Pharmaceuticals) and 320 mg of gentamycin were strung on No. 2 nonabsorbable suture and inserted into the wound bed. Rather than close the

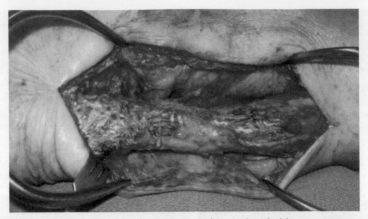

Fig. 2. Intraoperative photograph of AT repair with nonabsorbable suture mass.

site primarily, we used negative pressure wound therapy (NPWT) at 75 mm Hg for a mechanical leech effect. A well-padded sterile dressing was then applied from toes to knee with the addition of a plaster sugar tong and anterior bolster dressing maintaining the foot in gravity equinus.

In the interim between the first and second procedures, Gram stain results showed a few white blood cells but no organisms. The culture results showed no growth and the pathology report returned a diagnosis of ulceration with marked chronic inflammation and fibrosis.

SECOND SURGERY: RESTORATION OF PLANTARFLEXION

On initial inspection of the surgical site and removal of the antibiotic-impregnated PMMA beads, no signs of infection were appreciated. The skin edge about the lateral

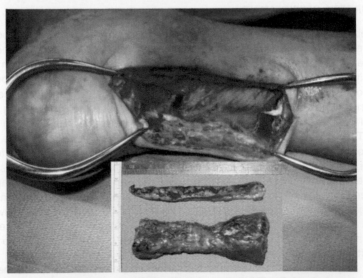

Fig. 3. Intraoperative photograph of the defect created following excision of 10-cm AT segment and overlying wound (inset).

portion of the incision was not viable, necessitating resection. The result of the skin resection ultimately prevented delayed primary closure. The wound was irrigated with 6 L of sterile saline via pulsed lavage. Intraoperatively, the AT defect was confirmed to be too large for primary end-to-end repair or secondary repair with advancement or rotational flap bridging using the gastrocnemius aponeurosis. Thus, we proceeded with transfer of the FHL and PB tendons to the calcaneus to restore plantarflexion tension. A description of this is outlined as follows.

An incision was placed over the lateral border of the foot about the base of the fifth metatarsal and carried deep to the level of the peroneal tendons. The PB and peroneus longus (PL) were sutured together with nonabsorbable sutures at this site. Then the PB was secured with a Krackow-type suture and severed proximal to the anastomosis. The tendon was then delivered to the posterior leg through the original incision, taking care to preserve as many of the perforating muscle vascular bundles as possible.

Next, the deep fascia of the leg was incised and the FHL muscle belly and tendon identified. We then performed a harvest of the FHL tendon at the medial arch through a secondary incision. We identified the conjoined tendons of the FHL and flexor digitorum longus at the Master Knot of Henry, secured the FHL with a Krackow-type suture, and then severed it proximal to the Master Knot (**Fig. 4**). Similar to retrieval of the PB tendon, we then delivered the FHL tendon through the posterior incision. The FHL tendon was passed through a transosseous tunnel made through the posterior calcaneal tuberosity from medial-to-lateral and was secured under tension with nonabsorbable suture to the PL tendon laterally. The redundant tendon was resected.

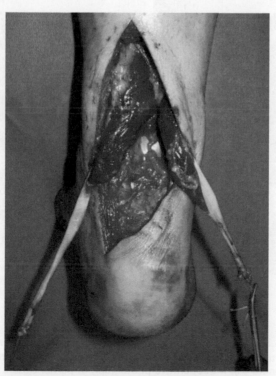

Fig. 4. Intraoperative photograph of harvested FHL and PB tendons.

The PB tendon was then brought from lateral-to-medial through a second transosseous tunnel and secured to the FHL tendon medially (**Fig. 5**A). This achieved a resting position of 15° of plantarflexion with dorsiflexion to −5° when moderate force was applied.

We noted a posterior calcaneal contour defect and this was concerning for eventual pressure necrosis of the overlying skin and thus we elected to pack this defect with an absorbable gelatin compressed sponge to achieve some degree of restoration of the defect. The FHL and PB muscle bellies were gently fanned out and sutured together to cover the deep tissues and tendons (**Fig. 5**B). The adjacent skin edges were brought to the muscle without tension. This left a wound defect the size of a silver dollar with a base consisting of the viable PB and FHL muscles (**Fig. 6**). As mentioned previously, primary closure would have proved difficult, so we again used NPWT at 75 mm Hg for a mechanical leech effect and a well-padded (including extra padding about the posterior heel and Achilles region) dressing was then applied from toes to knee with the addition of a plaster sugar tong and anterior bolster dressing to maintain the foot at 20° of plantarflexion.

THIRD SURGERY: CLOSURE

Four days later, we returned to the operating room for planned split-thickness skin graft (STSG) over the remaining wound according to the senior author's (TSR) protocol.[13] On removal of the dressing, we found the tendon transfer reconstruction of the

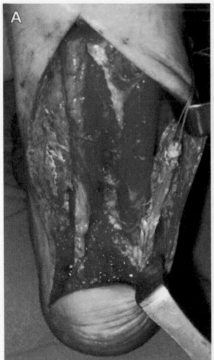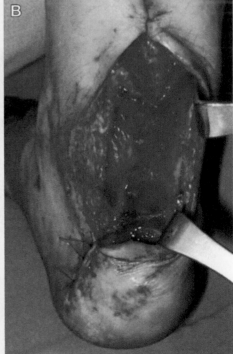

Fig. 5. Intraoperative photograph of final placement of transferred FHL and PB tendons through the calcaneus (*A*). Intraoperative photograph of partial closure over the FHL and PB tendons with myotendinous muscle fascia (*B*).

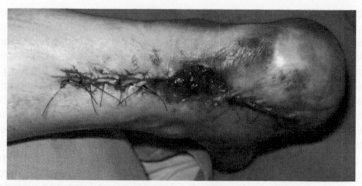

Fig. 6. Final closure with resultant skin defect and 100% muscular base.

AT had maintained its ability to plantarflex the foot. The skin edges appeared viable and well adhered to the surrounding edges of the muscular wound bed. The site was irrigated and then gently débrided to bleeding tissue and hemostasis obtained with gentle compression. The STSG was conveniently harvested from the patient's posterior central calf, which kept the donor site within the same postoperative dressing. We meshed the STSG in a 1.0:1.5 ratio, then transferred it to the operative site and secured it with multiple simple interrupted 3 to 0 chromic sutures (**Fig. 7**). A small section of reticulated foam was applied to the skin graft and secured with NPWT at 75 mm Hg with no pressure to the skin edges.

A well-padded sterile dressing was then applied from toes to knee with the addition of a plaster sugar tong and anterior bolster dressing maintaining the foot at gravity equinus to the lower leg.

REHABILITATION AND RECOVERY

The patient remained an inpatient at our institution for the entire course of the 3 operations. After the final procedure, he stayed in-house for an additional 4 days for pain control, planned discontinuation of the NPWT, and to participate in physical therapy to ensure his ability to remain non–weight bearing to the affected extremity. The patient was discharged on appropriate oral analgesics for postoperative pain and a muscle relaxant for muscle spasms about the operative lower leg. Furthermore, he followed our standard outpatient deep vein thrombosis prophylaxis protocol, which includes

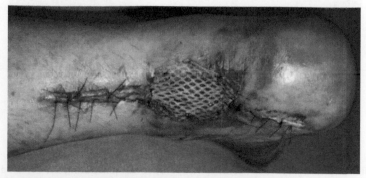

Fig. 7. STSG applied to the superficial defect for final closure.

aspirin 325 mg twice daily along with an anti-embolism stocking to the nonoperative lower leg, hourly mobility, and sustained hydration. He remained non–weight bearing in a modified Sir Robert Jones dressing reinforced with a plaster sugar tong splint with his foot in equinus for 8 weeks and then he was transitioned into a controlled-ankle motion boot with his ankle at 90°. At the 10-week mark, as the surgical sites were healed and the STSG had fully matured, the patient was allowed to begin limited weight bearing for transfers and short distance ambulation. After 15 weeks, he began a dedicated physical therapy routine to increase strength and improve plantarflexion about his ankle. Three weeks later, he was able to successfully complete heel raises and hypertrophy of the transferred tendons was noted on physical examination. An MRI was obtained after 6 months and revealed the transferred tendons and transosseous tunnels within the calcaneus to be free from infection and in good repair. The patient was last seen 20 months after the surgical procedures and was doing well (**Fig. 8**). The operative sites were stable to manual stress and the ankle joint demonstrated appropriate range of motion without abnormal instability. The patient had good active plantarflexion of the foot at the ankle joint and his resting tension was comparable to his contralateral limb. Furthermore, he was able to achieve 5° of dorsiflexion, which is the same as the contralateral limb.

Postoperative complications were limited to intermittent superficial wounding over the STSG site managed with physician-directed dressing changes according to the senior author's (TSR) protocol.[14] This was resolved with modified shoe heel counters to take pressure off of the cicatrix. Although he regained adequate ankle joint plantarflexion strength and was able to ambulate without difficulty, it was advised that he not return to either his former paper route or house-cleaning chores due to the complicated repair and high demands of these activities; the patient was amenable to these restrictions.

DISCUSSION

To our knowledge, there is no reported instance of concomitant transfer of the FHL and PB to reconstruct an AT. However, use of each tendon individually through a transosseous drill hole in the calcaneus to augment AT repair has been reported. Use of the PB through a transosseous drill hole in the calcaneus for AT rupture repair was originally described by Pérez-Teuffer[5] in 1974 when he passed the PB tendon through a transverse, transosseous drill hole in the calcaneus tuberosity and sutured it back onto the AT. He reported on 30 patients with AT ruptures repaired using his

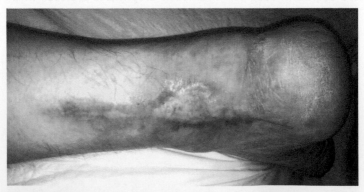

Fig. 8. Clinical photograph 20 months postoperative demonstrating well-healed surgical and STSG harvest sites.

technique, of which 28 had excellent and 2 had good outcomes with a mean follow-up of 5 years. The only reported complications involved 2 instances of delayed wound healing, both of which resolved uneventfully. In 1987, Turco and Spinella[6] described a modification of this technique by passing the PB tendon through the distal stump of the AT as opposed to the calcaneus, and this technique has been reproduced with good results.[7] A more recent study in 2013 by Tawari and colleagues[8] returned to the transosseous transfer approach, and reported on their modification of the Pérez-Teuffer[5] technique in 20 patients for acute AT ruptures. Although performed on acute rather than chronic ruptures, their results were similar, with a mean age of 41 years and a minimum follow-up of 18 months. They reported 85% good to excellent results and experienced 1 re-rupture, 1 superficial infection, 2 hypertrophic scars, and 3 patients who complained of hypoesthesia postoperatively.

Similar to the recruitment of the PB tendon, FHL transfer via a comparable approach has also been reported in the literature. Wapner and colleagues[9] first described this technique in 1993. It involved harvest of the FHL tendon distal to the Master Knot of Henry and subsequent tenodesis of the distal FHL stump to the nearby flexor digitorum longus tendon. They then gained exposure of the AT insertion and the posterior calcaneus and a series of 2 drill holes were made with the first placed just deep to the AT insertion, from dorsal-to-plantar in the middle of the calcaneal tuberosity, and then the second from medial-to-lateral, connecting with the first drill hole midway through the posterior calcaneus. The FHL tendon was then passed from proximal to distal through the bone tunnel and the transfer was completed by weaving the tendon through the remaining portion of the AT. They reported on their series of 7 patients with chronic AT ruptures. Three patients had undergone previous surgery before FHL reconstruction. The mean age was 52 years and the mean follow-up was 17 months. There were no postoperative complications and they noted simply that all patients experienced an insignificant loss in range of motion of the ankle and hallux, but all achieved satisfactory return to prior activities. Then, in 2010, Wegrzyn and colleagues[10] reported on their series of 11 patients with chronic AT rupture, who were treated by a modified FHL transfer involving a transosseous tunnel through the posterior calcaneus. Their modification of the original technique primarily involved a complete transverse tunnel through the posterior calcaneus and medial-to-lateral transfer of the FHL tendon, which was harvested at the Master Knot of Henry. Their patient demographics were similar, with a mean age of 44 years; however, they reported a longer mean follow-up of 6.6 years. Like Wapner and colleagues,[9] all patients presented with some loss of active range of motion at the hallux interphalangeal joint, but they noted none of their patients had subsequent hyperextension or any subjective complaints of weakness or decreased function during athletic activities. They also reported no complications encountered, aside from 1 temporary development of reflex sympathetic dystrophy. Others have also reported on the use of a transosseous tunnel through which to transfer the FHL tendon, including in a case report of reconstruction of bilateral xanthoma of the AT.[11]

Both transfers of the PB and FHL tendons have been reported with varying modifications of the previously mentioned techniques and have yielded good results. Again to our knowledge, there is no reported instance of concomitant transfer of the FHL and PB to reconstruct a chronically ruptured AT.

SUMMARY

Deep infection requiring the complete resection of the AT is rarely encountered. When this does occur, plantarflexion is compromised and in need of restoration. Any form of reconstruction undertaken should aim to restore as much of this lost strength as possible in a safe, reliable manner. However, limited options exist when managing catastrophic failure of an infected AT rupture repair. Use of allograft, xenograft, or synthetic products would be inappropriate in such a recently infected surgical site. We demonstrated the use of a local, double tendon transfer to restore the power and function of the AT. This technique successfully used a combined FHL and PB tendon transfer to restore adequate plantarflexion after complete loss of the AT due to infection. Although the patient was not able to return to more strenuous activities, his day-to-day activities were not restricted.

REFERENCES

1. Maffulli N. Rupture of the Achilles tendon. J Bone Joint Surg Am 1999;81(7): 1019–36.
2. Young JS, Sayana MK, McClelland D, et al. Peroneus brevis tendon transfer for delayed Achilles tendon ruptures. Tech Foot Ankle Surg 2005;4(3):143–7.
3. Ahluwalia R, Zourelidis C, Guo S, et al. Chronic sinus formation using non absorbable braided suture following open repair of Achilles tendon. Foot Ankle Surg 2013;19(2):e7–9.
4. Rosenzweig S, Azar FM. Open repair of acute Achilles tendon ruptures. Foot Ankle Clin 2009;14(4):699–709.
5. Pérez-Teuffer A. Traumatic rupture of the Achilles tendon: reconstruction by transplant and graft using the lateral peroneus brevis. Orthop Clin North Am 1974;5:89–93.
6. Turco V, Spinella AJ. Achilles tendon ruptures: peroneus brevis transfer. Foot Ankle 1987;7:253–9.
7. Pintore E, Barra V, Pintore R, et al. Peroneus brevis tendon transfer in neglected tears of the Achilles tendon. J Trauma 2001;50(1):71–8.
8. Tawari AA, Dhamangaonkar AA, Goregaonkar AB, et al. Augmented repair of degenerative tears of tendo Achilles using peroneus brevis tendon: early results. Malays Orthop J 2013;7(1):19–24.
9. Wapner KL, Pavlock GS, Hecht PJ, et al. Repair of chronic Achilles tendon rupture with flexor hallucis longus tendon transfer. Foot Ankle 1993;14(8):443–9.
10. Wegrzyn J, Luciani JF, Philippot R, et al. Chronic Achilles tendon rupture reconstruction using a modified flexor hallucis longus transfer. Int Orthop 2010;34(8): 1187–92.
11. Moroney PJ, Besse JL. Resection of bilateral massive Achilles tendon xanthomata with reconstruction using a flexor hallucis longus tendon transfer and Bosworth turndown flap: a case report and literature review. Foot Ankle Surg 2012;18(3):e25–8.
12. Schade VL, Roukis TS. The role of polymethylmethacrylate antibiotic–loaded cement in addition to debridement for the treatment of soft tissue and osseous infections of the foot and ankle. J Foot Ankle Surg 2010;49(1):55–62.
13. Roukis TS, Zgonis T. Skin grafting techniques for soft-tissue coverage of diabetic foot and ankle wounds. J Wound Care 2005;14(4):173–6.
14. Schade VL, Roukis TS. Use of a surgical preparation and sterile dressing change during office visit treatment of chronic foot and ankle wounds decreases the incidence of infection and treatment costs. Foot Ankle Spec 2008;1(3):147–54.

Complications of Tendon Surgery in the Foot and Ankle

Eric A. Barp, DPM[a,b,*], John G. Erickson, DPM[b]

KEYWORDS

- Tendon surgery • Complications • Diabetes • Tobacco • Achilles tendon
- Peroneal tendon

KEY POINTS

- With the exception of the Achilles tendon, little has been published on tendon healing and complications of tendon surgery in the foot and ankle.
- Complications of tendon surgery are often multifactorial, and their treatment should encompass that.
- A thorough history and physical examination minimizes the risk of complications, and provides a complete surgical plan.
- Tobacco use and uncontrolled diabetes significantly increase the rate of complications in tendon surgery of the foot and ankle.

INTRODUCTION

Tendon surgery in the foot and ankle is commonly performed for numerous pathologies. Although many of these procedures have reproducible positive results, occasionally the foot and ankle surgeon runs into a myriad of potential complications. These complications can lead to significant patient morbidity and mortality, especially if undertreated. Thus, it is imperative that the foot and ankle surgeon be well educated in the operative and nonoperative treatment options for these common complications.

Generally speaking, complications from tendon surgery originate from two sources: the patient or the surgeon. A patient's medical comorbidities and quality of tissue significantly impact their rate of healing and their risk for complications. Furthermore, the surgical plan and technique, as dictated by the surgeon, can also lead to increased

Disclosure Statement: The authors have nothing to disclose.
[a] The Iowa Clinic, 5950 University Avenue, West Des Moines, IA 50266, USA; [b] Unity Point Health, 1415 Woodland Avenue, #100, Des Moines, IA 50309, USA
* Corresponding author. The Iowa Clinic, 5950 University Avenue, West Des Moines, IA 50266.
E-mail address: ebarp@iowaclinic.com

risk of complications. As such, care must be taken to optimize all facets of the planned procedure to minimize the overall risk as much as possible. It is important to recognize the possibility of complications occurring despite perfect conditions and adequate preoperative planning.

For the purpose of this article, the focus first is on the common causes of general complications, and then on two specific groups of tendon procedures that are at a higher risk for complications: peroneal tendon and the Achilles tendon repairs.

RISK OF TOBACCO USE

The cardiopulmonary risks of tobacco use have been well established in medical literature. Recent studies show smoking to be a significant risk factor for delayed healing and nonunions in elective foot surgery,[1] ankle fractures, and ankle and subtalar arthrodesis. The effect of smoking on wound healing has also been shown throughout the literature; however, specific studies are lacking regarding tendon healing in the foot and ankle. Fortunately, there are a few studies throughout the general orthopedic literature that are applicable and can help guide clinicians.

Bruggeman and colleagues[2] performed an analysis on wound complications in patients with open repair of Achilles tendon ruptures. They retrospectively reviewed 167 cases of open Achilles tendon repairs. Their data show smokers had a 38% chance of wound complications compared with 7.8% chance of wound complications in nonsmokers. Other than smoking, only the use of steroids and being female were found to have a statistically significant effect on wound healing complications. Unfortunately, other complications of Achilles tendon surgery were not included in this study.

Sorensen and colleagues[3] published a study in 2003 looking at the effects of abstaining from smoking on incisional wound infections. In their study, they compared 48 smokers with 30 patients who had never smoked, and followed them for 15 weeks. The smokers consumed 20 cigarettes per day for the first week before being randomized into three groups: (1) continuous smoking, (2) absence of smoking with nicotine patch, and (3) absence of smoking with placebo patch. An elliptical incision was then made just lateral to the sacrum, which was sutured and followed throughout its healing process. Incisions were performed at the end of the first week and at 4, 8, and 12 weeks after randomization. The wound infection rate in smokers was 12% compared with 2% in nonsmokers. The rate of wound infections significantly dropped in the placebo and nicotine patch groups at 4, 8, and 12 weeks. This study suggests that cessation 1 month before surgery may help decrease the risk of incisional wound healing complications. This study also suggests that nicotine replacement patches may not hinder healing as previously thought. There have been other studies published on this topic, but the results further solidify that the exact mechanism of how smoking inhibits wound healing is complicated and multifaceted, extending beyond just the effects of the nicotine alone.

Moller and colleagues[4] performed a retrospective analysis of 825 patients undergoing hip or knee arthroplasty. They compared 454 nonsmokers with 232 smokers while comparing wound healing complications, cardiopulmonary complications, intensive care requirements, and length of hospital stay. Smokers were found to have a higher risk for developing wound complications and also had a higher rate of admissions to the critical care unit, generally for pulmonary complications. Mallon and colleagues[5] performed a retrospective analysis of 224 patients with an open rotator cuff repair. They had 95 smokers and 129 nonsmokers. They found that nonsmokers had significantly less pain compared with smokers. They also found that smokers had a worse preoperative and post operative score than their nonsmoking counterparts.

Santiago-Torres and coworkers[6] performed a meta-analysis looking at the effects of smoking on rotator cuff and glenoid labrum surgery. Ten studies met inclusion criteria, and they found that smoking had a negative influence on rotator cuff clinical outcomes and was associated with decreased healing rates in rotator cuff tears. The authors of this study make no attempt to extrapolate the data globally to all tendon surgery; however, the tenuous blood supply to the rotator cuff is not unlike the blood supply to the distal tendons in the lower extremities. At the completion of their study, the authors recommend surgeons to encourage smoking cessation before performing surgery.

In 2008, Walker and colleagues[7] published a study looking the effect of preoperative counseling on smoking patterns in patients undergoing surgery. They had 97 patients undergo surgery during their study period, of these 25 were recorded as smokers. Sixteen of these patients stated that they stopped smoking preoperatively, whereas four patients stated that they decreased their nicotine consumption. All of the smokers in this study stated that they were unaware of the negative effects of smoking on healing foot surgery. This study should further encourage the surgeon that adequate patient education in smoking cessation is beneficial and effective in 64% of patients.

Although there currently are no studies in the literature specifically looking at the effects of tobacco use on tendon healing in foot and ankle surgery, there is still sufficient evidence to guide recommendations and therapy. As shown, there is a substantial body of evidence specifically showing an increased risk of wound healing complications with tobacco use. Although the exact mechanism is still debated, Campanile and colleagues[8] suggest that the outcomes are a cumulative effect of tissue hypoxia, vessel vasoconstriction, and inhibition of cellular oxidative metabolism, and potentially a few additional pathways. Conversely, there has been some evidence that hypoxia can actually lead to angiogenesis and theoretically increase healing rates of wounds. The clinical applications of these studies are extremely controversial. The medical and scientific community still has a lot of ground to cover to fully understand this process; however, currently there is sufficient evidence to support and encourage the abstinence of tobacco starting a month before surgery, and extending through the healing process.

RISK OF TENDON SURGERY IN PATIENTS WITH DIABETES

Much has been published regarding the increased risk for postsurgical complications in the diabetic patient population. Diabetes mellitus continues to be a major health problem in the United States affecting 25.8 million people,[9] and this number is only expected to grow in the coming years.[10] Most of the clinical literature has focused more on incisional wound healing in the foot and ankle, then tendon healing specifically. The scientific community has produced multiple studies in rat models that help in understanding the pathologic processes specifically related to tendon healing.

Lehto and colleagues[11] published a study in 1996, examining the predictors of lower extremity amputation in patients with non–insulin-dependent diabetes. In this study, they followed 1044 patients for a 7-year period of time. At the conclusion of the study they found that there was dose-response relationship between plasma glucose/ HbA_{1c}, and the risk for amputation. This risk remained even after adjusting for other cardiovascular risk factors. Other important predictors for amputation were peripheral neuropathy, bilateral absence of Achilles tendon reflexes, absence of vibration sense, and absent peripheral pulses. Aronow and colleagues[12] found a correlation between increased HbA_{1c} and severity of peripheral arterial disease, both of which have been found to be independent risk factors for wound complications and subsequent amputation. These risk factors need to be respected when considering any surgical procedure.

Humphers and colleagues[13] published a study in 2014 attempting to determine the risk of postoperative infection after foot and ankle surgery, relative to the increasing HbA_{1c}. The goal of their study was to question the guidelines published by the American Diabetes Association, who state that elective surgery should be avoided in patients whose HbA_{1c} is greater than 7%. Humphers' study found that the average A1C of patients who experienced complications was 8.26%, versus those that did not experience complications, who's HbA_{1c} was 7.17%. In their study a significant increase in infection rate occurred between 7.3% and 9.8%. This suggests that an HbA_{1c} of 7% may be too strict of a guideline, and the surgeon may consider expanding this to 8%.

Wukich and colleagues[14] published a prospective study in 2014 evaluating the risk of infection after foot and ankle surgery. They looked at 2060 consecutive surgical cases, and compared patients with diabetes with patients with neuropathy, with respective control groups. The overall infection rate was 3.1%. Complications of patients with uncontrolled diabetes had a 7.25-fold increase. It is also important to note that patients without diabetes with peripheral neuropathy also had a 4.72-fold increase. Although increased hemoglobin glycosylation increased the risk significantly, it is important to realize that a similar increase was seen in patients with neuropathy without diabetes.

Although the exact mechanism of tendon derangement in patients with diabetes is not completely understood, recent studies have shown that the damage is caused by an excess of advanced glycation end products. These advanced glycation end products can form a covalent cross-link within collagen fibers, which then causes alterations in their structure and affects their ability to function. A study of diabetic mouse tendons performed by Connizzo and colleagues[15] in 2014 showed that the mechanical properties of diabetic tendons were altered as compared with nondiabetic tendons. Their study found that diabetic mice had a statistically significant difference in the cross-sectional area, stiffness, and response to load as compared with nondiabetic mouse tendons. This difference was attributed primarily to collagen fiber realignment.

Similar changes in the Achilles tendon have been described in humans using MRI and ultrasound modalities. One such study was published in 2014 by de Jonge and colleagues.[16] In this article, ultrasound was used to compare the structure of the Achilles tendon in patients with and without diabetes. Abnormal sonographic appearance of the tendon was present in patients with diabetes more frequently than their control subjects. It should be noted, however, that increased body mass index was also found to be associated with these structural changes. A similar study was performed by Abate and colleagues in 2014.[17] In this study they found that patients with diabetes were more likely to have asymptomatic sonographic abnormalities than patients without diabetes; specifically, there was a higher rate of Achilles enthesiopathy.

In 2014, Mohsenifar and colleagues[18] looked at the healing rate of tenotomised Achilles tendons in diabetic rats. They found that the diabetic tendons had significantly less elasticity and stress tensile load. The level of inflammation was higher in the diabetic rats, and the level of fibrosis was significantly lower than in the control group. They postulate that these findings suggest a slower rate of healing in patients with diabetes as compared with patients without diabetes. A similar study was published in 2012 by Egemen and colleagues,[19] which compared streptozotocin-induced diabetic rats with healthy rats. After 3 days, both Achilles tendons were transected and subsequently repaired. The rats were then euthanized at 2, 4, and 6 weeks and the limbs were mechanically tested. The results of this study showed that the diabetic rats had a statistically significant lower peak force for failure at each phase of testing.

They also found a significantly smaller amount of fibroblast proliferation and lymphocyte infiltration in the diabetic rats. They conclude that patients with diabetes should be followed very closely postoperatively, to ensure that subsequent rerupture does not occur.

Several articles have been published in the literature looking at the effects of diabetes in rotator cuff repairs. One such article was published by Cho and colleagues[20] in 2015, where they set out to compare the outcomes of arthroscopic rotator cuff repair in patients with diabetes versus without diabetes. Postoperative MRI scans were used to assess the integrity of their repair. In doing so, 14.4% of the patients without diabetes and 35.9% of the patients with diabetes had some degree of retearing. A total of 43.2% of patients with diabetes who's A1C was greater than 7% experienced a retear, compared with 25.9% of patients whose A1C was less than 7%.

It is important for the foot and ankle surgeon to understand the increased risk of complications in the diabetic patient population. As discussed, these patients frequently have multiple comorbidities that individually and collectively increase the risk of tendon rupture, incisional wound healing, and amputation. Although there are no studies in the literature, to our knowledge, that have been published on the effects of diabetes on tendon healing in foot and ankle surgery, we are able to extrapolate data from rat models and the general orthopedic literature to support our decision making. These patients must be handled carefully, progressed through the recovery phase with caution, and medically optimized before elective procedures. This should include achieving an HbA_{1c} below 8, ensuring adequate blood flow, weight loss, and their ability to comply with postoperative protocols. If the surgeon is able to achieve these goals, one can effectively reduce the risk of complications for these patients, although they will likely remain at an increased risk as compared with their counterparts with no diabetes.

COMPLICATIONS IN PERONEAL TENDON SURGERY

Peroneal tendon pathology is commonly seen by foot and ankle surgeons; however, its exact prevalence in society remains unknown. DiGiovanni and coworkers[21] found that 25% to 77% of patients with lateral ankle instability also had some level of peroneal tendon pathology. Complications of the surgical treatment of these pathologies include infection, dehiscence, weakness, sural neuritis and recurrence. The rate of complications has yet to be established in the literature. Most complications of surgical correction of peroneal pathology are secondary to inappropriate procedure selection secondary to inadequately diagnosing the entirety of the pathology. In 1998 Krause and Brodsky[22] proposed a treatment algorithm for peroneal tendon tears. They recommend direct repair of tendons that have less than 50% of their cross-sectional area involved in the tear. If the tear encompasses greater than 50% of the tendon, they recommend performing a tenodesis. Since its publication, this simple guideline has become extremely popular among foot and ankle surgeons, and has helped guide intraoperative decision making.

Although complications of peroneal tendon surgery are rare, they certainly do occur. Frequently these patients are worked-up with an MRI preoperatively to evaluate the extent of the pathology. Although MRI has been shown to be sensitive for peroneal pathologies, it can frequently underestimate the involvement of the tear, or miss a concomitant tear in the peroneus longus tendon. If a surgeon relies too heavily on the MRI to evaluate the extent of the pathology, they place the patient at an increased risk for surgical complications secondary to undertreatment. Peroneal tendon tears certainly can be acute in nature; however, they are much more frequently degenerative in nature. This degeneration of the tendon can frequently leave the tendon frayed and the surgeon must determine if the remaining tendon is viable and able to perform the task required of it. If the peroneal tendon is unable to be tubulerized, or end-to-end repair is unable to be achieved, the surgeon needs to have several contingency plans prepared. These contingency plans can and should include tendon transfers, tenodesis, or allograft tendon repairs.

Although a thorough discussion on treatment options is beyond the scope of this article, a brief discussion on treatment decision making is merited. Complications commonly arise when validated treatment algorithms are not followed. One such algorithm was published by Redfern and Myerson[23] for the treatment of concomitant peroneal tendon tears in 2004. They treated a total of 29 feet with good results across all levels of pathology. They divided these patients into three classes: type 1 injuries had both tendons grossly intact, type 2 had one tendon torn and the other was "usable," type 3 had both tendons torn/unusable, type 3A had no excursion of the proximal muscle, and type 3B had excursion of the proximal muscle. Type 1 and 2 injuries were repaired as described by Krause and Brodsky. Type 3A injuries required a tendon transfer, because allograft was unlikely to be successful in the absence of muscle excursion. Type 3B injuries were reconstructed with allograft either as a primary procedure, or staged with a silicon rod implant if exorbitant scar tissue was present in the wound bed.

Failure to recognize the entirety of the deformity is another major cause of complications. To ensure the best potential for a successful operation, it is imperative to address all concomitant structural deformities. The previously mentioned article by Redfern and Myerson is one example of a study where they found that 21 of 28 patients had concomitant deformities: 12 of 28 patients had subjective lateral ankle instability, eight of which had objective lateral ankle instability; 6 of 28 had hindfoot varus; and 3 of 28 had a cavovarus deformity. Recurrent subluxation of the peroneal tendons can also be secondary to a convex, or flat, peroneal groove on the posterior aspect of the fibula. Although this structure is formed by fibrocartilage, and is not osseous in nature, its presence intraoperatively should be confirmed and addressed if determined necessary. Several options have been described in the literature including anatomic repairs that focus on recreating the superior peroneal retinaculum, bone-block procedures,[24,25] groove-deepening procedures,[26] and distal fibular reaming.[27]

Tenodesis of the peroneal tendons has been shown to be effective, if performed correctly. The tenotomies should be performed 3 to 4 cm proximal and 5 cm distal to the fibular tip to prevent fibular impingement. Furthermore, a prominent peroneal tubercle can cause significant damage and fraying to the peroneal tendons. If this structure is enlarged, it should be excised at the time of surgical correction of the tendon pathology to prevent recurrence. Another common complication of peroneal tendon surgery is sural neuritis, which is discussed as it pertains to Achilles tendon complications.

COMPLICATIONS IN ACHILLES TENDON SURGERY

The literature has a substantial number of publications focusing on the complications of Achilles tendon surgery. This is largely caused by the high rate of Achilles tendon ruptures, as high as 18 in 100,000 males. Ruptures most frequently occur in the watershed zone located 2 to 6 cm proximal to the distal attachment. The surgical treatment in this region has been plagued with complications in wound healing. Furthermore, the Achilles tendon is at an increased risk of rerupture secondary to amount of force that transferred through the tendon with every step. Much has been published on surgical versus nonsurgical therapy for Achilles tendon ruptures. Nonoperative treatment has the benefits of less ankle joint stiffness, less calf atrophy, fewer adhesions, and lower risk of thrombophlebitis as compared with surgical correction. Nonsurgical therapy, however, has an increased risk for lengthening the Achilles tendon leading to decreased strength, and potentially a calcaneal gate. There is also an increased risk of rerupture in nonsurgically treated Achilles tendon ruptures.[28,29] Other complications of surgical treatment include deep and superficial wound infections, skin and tendon necrosis, fistulas, scar adhesion, sural nerve damage, decreased ankle motion, over-lengthening of the tendon, deep venous thrombosis (DVT), and pulmonary embolus.

One of the most frequent complications of Achilles tendon surgery are wound heal-ing complications, including incisional dehiscence, deep and superficial infections, adhesions, and scar irritation. Wong and colleagues[30] found minor wound complica-tions occurred in 12.3% after open repair; this was decreased to 4.9% with percuta-neous techniques and 0.5% with conservative therapy. Khan and colleagues[29] found that early mobilization significantly reduced the risk of wound healing complications, specifically adhesions, in the surgical and conservative groups. The study by Brugge-man and coworkers[2] looked at 164 patients with wound complications in 10.4% of the patients. A secondary analysis of these patients found that tobacco use, steroid use, and being female significantly increased the risk of these complications. Interestingly, presence of diabetes, increased body mass index, age, and time to surgery did not lead to increased risk in wound healing.

The risk of wound healing complications can be diminished by adhering to several fundamental techniques. The surgeon should use gentle retraction with a "no-touch technique"; this is frequently performed with suture at the incision. The suture is then held with a hemostat or temporarily sutured to the surrounding skin. A full-thickness incision should be used to reduce the risk of partial wound necrosis and fail-ure. This incision should be made respecting the angiosomes to the posterior heel as described by Attinger and coworkers,[31] but also respecting the variability of the loca-tion of the sural nerve. Assuming the patient has patent tibial and peroneal arteries, the incision should be made either midline or just medial to the midline. Furthermore, the surgeon should diligently close the paratenon at the conclusion of the case. This repair decreases the risk of adhesion formation surrounding the Achilles tendon; but it also functions as an additional layer of soft tissue over the repaired Achilles tendon in the event of incisional dehiscence.

Overlengthening of the Achilles tendon is an important cause of morbidity and mor-tality following Achilles tendon repair. This can be avoided if the surgeon adheres to several principles while performing the repair. A locking suture, as described by Krackow and coworkers[32] or one of its modifications, should be used to prevent give within the suture construct. The ankle should be placed in plantar flexion at the time of repair. Note that the musculotendon unit continues to stretch postoperatively, especially in chronic ruptures. If an overlengthened Achilles tendon occurs, the treat-ment and recovery is quite difficult to manage. Nonoperatively focus should be placed on strengthening the secondary plantarflexors. Proprioceptive therapy and end range of motion (ROM) plantar flexion strengthening should be stressed. Some support ex-ists for Achilles tendon shortening procedures including Bohnsack and colleagues,[33] who performed the procedure on eight patients. All eight continued to show decreased strength in plantarflexion, but the patients all had improved gate, improved activity level, and decreased pain.

Sural neuritis is another common complication following surgical correction of Achil-les tendon ruptures. The sural nerve is a sensory branch of the tibial nerve that descends from between the heads of the gastrocnemius and crosses the lateral border of the Achilles tendon, approximately 9.8 cm proximal to its insertion. The nerve then travels just lateral to the Achilles tendon with the small saphenous vein, approximately 17.5 mm lateral to the calcaneal insertion of the Achilles tendon. Damage to this nerve perioperatively can lead to long-term neuritis and in some patients can lead to complex regional pain syndrome. Rates of sural neuritis in the literature range from 0% to 20% with open Achilles tendon procedures. Nistor's[34] study had a high complication rate of 20%; however, seven of the nine complications used a lateral incision. As such, a lateral approach should be avoided. Lo and colleagues[35] reviewed 701 cases and found that the overall rate of sural neuritis was 6%. Lim and colleagues[36] found that 7 of 66 patients had preoperative sural neuritis implying that the nerve was injured at the time of injury. Studies of sural neuritis in percutaneous procedures range from 3% to 40%[37] and mini-open or minimally invasive techniques average 9.2%.[38] Treatment of sural neuritis is difficult and prolonged. Some steps can be taken to reduce the risk of sural neuritis, including limiting the amount of deep closure and not applying an overly tight compressive dressing. If the nerve is inadvertently ligated in surgery, it should be buried deep within to peroneal muscles to prevent formation of a stump neuroma and reduce postoperative pain.

The development of complex regional pain syndrome has been sparsely described following surgery on the Achilles tendon; however, the risk is higher if a patient continues to have sural neuritis postoperatively. To our knowledge, only two cases of complex regional pain syndrome secondary to Achilles tendon surgery have been described in the literature. The first was from an Achilles tendon repair that was performed percutaneous and the second was performed using external fixation in the proximal portion of the tendon and distally to the calcaneus.[39,40] Complex regional pain syndrome presents as pain out of proportion with swelling and vasomotor instability. This swelling and decreased active ROM secondary to pain leads to significant joint stiffness and contracture. Type 1 complex regional pain syndrome, formally known as reflex sympathetic dystrophy, is secondary to a global injury, whereas type 2, formally known as causalgia, is theorized to be secondary to direct nerve injury. Achilles tendon ruptures and subsequent repair place patients at a theoretically increased risk level because both pathways can be initiated. Current evidence best supports use of physiotherapy for treatment of either type of complex regional pain syndrome.

The true prevalence of DVT after Achilles tendon surgery is difficult to quantify, because most DVTs are asymptomatic and presumably go undiagnosed. Symptomatic DVTs were included as part of the study by Lo and coworkers,[35] where they found only 1 symptomatic DVT in 701 patients treated operatively and 4 out of 248 nonsurgically treated patients. Lassen and colleagues[41] performed a double-blind placebo controlled trial in 440 patients to study the effects of subcutaneous reviparin. The patients all had lower extremity trauma, either an Achilles tendon rupture or an ankle fracture, which required them to be casted for at least 5 weeks. Surgical therapy versus conservative therapy was not included as part of their analysis. The patients were then examined with an ultrasound at 1 week postinjury and at the completion of the cast therapy. Nineteen percent of the placebo control group had a DVT by the completion of the study, whereas only 9% of the treatment group developed a DVT.

Discrepancies between the recommendations produced by different governing bodies add confusion to the prophylaxis debate. The American Association of Chest Physicians recommend against prophylaxis, whereas the Cochrane review and National Institute for Clinical Excellence, in the United Kingdom, both recommend routine prophylaxis with low-molecular-weight heparin. A recent Clinical Consensus

Statement has been published by the American College of Foot and Ankle Surgeons who state that DVT prophylaxis for prolonged immobilization, with and without foot and ankle surgery, should not be performed routinely. They elaborate and place the responsibility on the surgeon to stratify the risk of each individual patient taking into account personal history of DVT or pulmonary embolism, active or recent cancer, hypercoagulability, and prolonged lower extremity immobilization. Secondary risk factors were described as obesity, advanced age, oral contraceptive pill/hormone-replacement therapy use, family history of DVT, varicose veins, higher injury severity score, multiple medical comorbidities, hospitalization, bed rest, and general anesthesia. They also recommend low-molecular-weight heparin for therapy beginning 12 to 24 hours postinjury, or postoperatively, and continued throughout the period of immobilization. Furthermore, they stress the importance of decreasing the risk of thrombotic events by using multimodal therapy including chemical prophylaxis, sequential compression devices, compression hose, and early mobilization when possible.

The risk of rerupture of the Achilles tendon has been well studied in the current literature, as investigators continue to debate the superiority of surgical versus nonsurgical treatment of this pathology. A complete synopsis of this debate is beyond the scope of this article. Recent studies have attempted to delineate a difference between surgical therapy and nonoperative therapy with early ROM in a functional brace. However, many of these studies fail to incorporate the postoperative therapy and effectiveness of early ROM after surgical correction. In short, the risk of rerupture after surgery ranges from 0% to 3.5%. The meta-analysis by Soroceanu and coworkers[42] found that surgically treated patients had 15.8% greater chance of other complications; however, they did not differentiate between major and minor complications. They also found that surgically treated patients returned to work almost 3 weeks sooner than nonsurgically treated patients.

Proper suture technique needs to be used to ensure the strongest repair possible. Watson and colleagues[43] in 1995, found that a locking stitch, as described by Krackow and coworkers,[32] was superior to previously described suture techniques. New modifications of this technique have been described, which may show continued improvement, but additional studies need to be performed to validate their use. One such modification is the "gift box" technique as described by Labib and colleagues[44] in 2009. Initial studies have shown that a simple modification increased the mean force to failure from 81N with a standard Krackow technique, to 168N. This improvement has been postulated to be secondary a combination of two factors: first the knots are moved out of the defect site effectively reducing the risk of knot failure, and second this modification allows for four strands to cross the defect site rather than two strands.

Furthermore, preservation of the blood supply to the tendon is crucial to the prevention of rerupture. The central aspect of the Achilles tendon, from 2 to 6 cm proximal to its insertion in the calcaneus, has been described as a watershed zone. The primary blood flow to the tendon is supplied through the musculotendon junction and from the calcaneal insertion. The vascularity to the watershed zone is reinforced by a vascular network on the ventral aspect of the tendon; as such, dissection in this area should be minimized.

If the rupture occurred in the presence of a systemic disease (ie, gout or hyperparathyroidism) then these conditions need to be addressed further by the patient's primary care provider. Additionally, if the patient has decreased vascular perfusion secondary to peripheral arterial disease, then this needs to be addressed by a vascular surgeon or an interventional cardiologist that is familiar with treatment of lower extremity occlusive arterial disease.

When complications are encountered intraoperatively, the surgeon must have a full understanding of alternative means to address the deformity. Maffulli and Ajis[45] published a review in 2008 that looked at the treatment of chronic Achilles tendon ruptures. They also recommended that end-to-end repair of the defect was possible if the defect was less than 2.5 cm. In this article, they also provide a comprehensive review of treatment options for Achilles tendon ruptures, including V-Y tendon alignments,[46,47] turndown flaps,[48,49] peroneus brevis autograft,[50] flexor digitorum longus autografts,[51] flexor halluces longus autografts,[52] gracilis autografts,[53] facia lata autografts,[54] allografts, synthetic grafts, and minimally invasive techniques. Currently there are insufficient data to compare each of these procedures; but a crucial component to managing intraoperative complications is having multiple contingency plans available to the surgeon.

SUMMARY

It is imperative that the foot and ankle surgeon be well aware of the most frequent complications associated with the procedures being performed. A thorough history and physical examination protects the surgeon and patient from many avoidable complications. The surgeon must address the entire patient and foot structure, not just the obvious pathology. In many cases, these patients may require treatment from other specialties to ensure that they are optimized for healing prior proceeding with elective surgical procedures. Furthermore, a well prepared surgeon has multiple contingency plans available while in the operative theater, so as not to be caught off guard when the unforeseen occurs. Lastly, patient education should not be minimized. This is an important part of the process, allowing the patient to become their own advocate. Informing the patient how their decisions affect the potential outcome of their surgical procedures has been shown to be effective.

REFERENCES

1. Krannitz KW, Fong HW, Fallat LM, et al. The effect of cigarette smoking on radiographic bone healing after elective foot surgery. J Foot Ankle Surg 2009;48(5): 525–7.
2. Bruggeman N, Turner N, Dahm D, et al. Wound complications after open Achilles tendon repair: an analysis of risk factors. Clin Orthop Relat Res 2004;427:63–6.
3. Sorensen LT, Karlsmark T, Gottrup F. Abstinence from smoking reduces incisional wound infection: a randomized controlled trial. Ann Surg 2003;238:1–5.
4. Moller A, Pedersen T, Villebro N, et al. Effects of smoking on early complications after elective orthopaedic surgery. J Bone Joint Surg Br 2003;85:178–81.
5. Mallon W, Misamore G, Snead D, et al. The impact of preoperative smoking habits on the results of rotator cuff repair. J Shoulder Elbow Surg 2004;13:129–32.
6. Santiago-Torres J, Flanigan DC, Butler RB, et al. The effect of smoking on rotator cuff and glenoid labrum surgery: a systematic review. Am J Sports Med 2015;43:745.
7. Walker NM, Morris SA, Cannon LB. The effect of pre-operative counselling on smoking patterns in patients undergoing forefoot surgery. Foot Ankle Surg 2009;15:86–9.
8. Campanile G, Hautmann G, Lotti T. Cigarette smoking, wound healing and face lift. Clin Dermatol 1998;16:575–8.
9. Centers for Disease Control and Prevention. National diabetes fact sheet: national estimates and general information. 2011. Available at: http://www.cdc.gov/diabetes/pubs/factsheet11.htm. Accessed October 8, 2013.

10. Mokdad AH, Bowman BA, Ford ES, et al. The continuing epidemics of obesity and diabetes in the United States. JAMA 2001;286(10):1195–200.
11. Lehto S, Pyorala K, Rönnemaa T, et al. Risk factors predicting lower extremity amputations in patients with NIDDM. Diabetes Care 1996;6:607–12.
12. Aronow WS, Ahn C, Weiss MB, et al. Relation of increased hemoglobin A1c levels to severity of peripheral arterial disease in patients with diabetes mellitus. Am J Cardiol 2007;99:1468–9.
13. Humphers J, Shibuya N, Fluhman BL, et al. The impact of glycosylated hemoglobin and diabetes mellitus on postoperative wound healing complications and infection following foot and ankle surgery. J Am Podiatr Med Assoc 2014; Jun 24. [Epub ahead of print].
14. Wukich DK, Crim BE, Frykberg RG, et al. Neuropathy and poorly controlled diabetes increase the rate of surgical site infection after foot and ankle surgery. J Bone Joint Surg Am 2014;96:832–9.
15. Connizzo BK, Bhatt PR, Liechty KW, et al. Diabetes alters mechanical properties and collagen fiber re-alignment in multiple mouse tendons. Ann Biomed Eng 2014;42:1880–8.
16. de Jonge S, Rozenberg R, Vieyra B, et al. Achilles tendons in people with type 2 diabetes show mildly compromised structure: an ultrasound tissue characterization study. Br J Sports Med 2015;1–5.
17. Abate M, Salini V, Antinolfi P, et al. Ultrasound morphology of the Achilles in asymptomatic patients with and without diabetes. Foot Ankle Int 2014;35:44–9.
18. Mohsenifar Z, Feridoni MJ, Bayat M, et al. Histological and biomechanical analysis of the effects of streptozotocin-induced type one diabetes mellitus on healing of tenotomised Achilles tendons in rats. Foot Ankle Surg 2014;20:186–91.
19. Egemen O, Ozkaya O, Ozturk MB, et al. The biomechanical and histological effects of diabetes on tendon healing: experimental study in rats. J Hand Microsurg 2012;4:60–4.
20. Cho NS, Moon SC, Jeon JW, et al. The influence of diabetes mellitus on clinical and structural outcomes after arthroscopic rotator cuff repair. Am J Sports Med 2015;43(4):991–7.
21. DiGiovanni BF, Fraga CJ, Cohen BE, et al. Associated injuries found in chronic lateral ankle instability. Foot Ankle Int 2000;21:809–15.
22. Krause JO, Brodsky JW. Peroneus brevis tendon tears: pathophysiology, surgical reconstruction and clinical results. Foot Ankle Int 1998;19:271–9.
23. Redfern D, Myerson M. The management of concomitant tears of the peroneus longus and brevis tendons. Foot Ankle Int 2004;25:695–707.
24. Kelly RE. An operation for the chronic dislocation of the peroneal tendons. Br J Surg 1920;7:502–4.
25. Watson-Jones R. Fractures of joint injuries. 4th edition. Baltimore (MD): Williams & Wilkins; 1956.
26. Zoellner G, Clancy W. Recurrent dislocation of the peroneal tendon. J Bone Joint Surg Am 1979;61:292–4.
27. Mendicino RW, Orsini RC, Whitman SE, et al. Fibular groove deepening for recurrent peroneal subluxation. J Foot Ankle Surg 2001;40:252–63.
28. Soma CA, Mandelbaum BR. Repair of acute Achilles tendon rupture. Orthop Clin North Am 1995;26:239–47.
29. Khan RJ, Fick D, Keogh A, et al. Treatment of acute Achilles tendon ruptures: a meta-analysis of randomized, controlled trials. J Bone Joint Surg Am 2005;87:2201–10.
30. Wong J, Barrass V, Maffulli N. Quantitative review of operative and non-operative management of Achilles tendon ruptures. Am J Sports Med 2002;30:565–75.

31. Attinger CE, Evans KK, Bulan E, et al. Angiosomes of the foot and ankle and clinical implications for limb salvage: reconstruction, incisions, and revascularization. Plast Reconstr Surg 2006;117:261S–93S.

32. Krackow KA, Thomas SC, Jones LC. A new stitch for ligament-tendon fixation. J Bone Joint Surg Am 1986;68:764–6.

33. Bohnsack M, Ruhmann O, Kirshc L, et al. Surgical shortening of the Achilles tendon for correction of elongation following healed conservatively treated Achilles tendon rupture. Z Orthop Ihre Grenzgeb 2000;138:501–5.

34. Nistor L. Surgical and nonsurgical treatment of Achilles tendon rupture. A prospective randomized study. J Bone Joint Surg Am 1981;63:394–9.

35. Lo IK, Kirkley A, Nonweiler B, et al. Operative versus non-operative treatment of acute Achilles tendon ruptures: a quantitative review. Clin J Sport Med 1997;7: 207–11.

36. Lim J, Dalal R, Waseem M. Percutaneous vs open repair of the ruptured Achilles tendon—a prospective randomized controlled study. Foot Ankle Int 2001;22: 559–68.

37. Molloy A, Wood E. Complications of the treatment of Achilles tendon ruptures. Foot Ankle Clin N Am 2009;14:745–59.

38. Lansdaal JR, Goslings JC, Reichart M, et al. The results of 163 Achilles tendon ruptures treated by a minimally invasive surgical technique and functional after treatment. Injury 2007;38:839–44.

39. Webb JM, Bannister GC. Percutaneous repair of the ruptured tendoachillis. J Bone Joint Surg Br 1999;81:877–80.

40. Nada A. Rupture of the calcaneal tendon. Treatment by external fixation. J Bone Joint Surg Br 1985;67:449–53.

41. Lassen MR, Borris LC, Nakov RL. Use of low molecular weight heparin reviparin to prevent deep-vein thrombosis after leg injury requiring immobilization. N Engl J Med 2002;347:726–30.

42. Soroceanu A, Sidhwa F, Aarabi S, et al. Surgical versus nonsurgical treatment of acute Achilles tendon rupture; a meta-analysis of randomized trials. J Bone Joint Surg Am 2012;94:2136–43.

43. Watson TW, Jurist KA, Yang KH, et al. The strength of Achilles tendon repair: an in vivo study of the biomechanical behavior in human cadaver tendons. Foot Ankle 1995;16:191–5.

44. Labib SA, Rolf R, Dacus R, et al. The "Giftbox" repair of the Achilles tendon: a modification of the Krackow technique. Foot Ankle Int 2009;30:410–4.

45. Maffulli N, Ajis A. Management of chronic ruptures of the Achilles tendon. J Bone Joint Surg Am 2008;90:1348–60.

46. Abraham E, Pankovich AM. Neglected rupture of the Achilles tendon. Treatment by V-Y tendinous flap. J Bone Joint Surg Am 1975;57:253–5.

47. Leitner A, Voigt C, Rahmanzadeh R. Treatment of extensive aseptic defects in old Achilles tendon ruptures: methods and case reports. Foot Ankle 1992;13: 176–80.

48. Christensen I. Rupture of the Achilles tendon; analysis of 57 cases. Acta Chir Scand 1953;106:50–60.

49. Mulier T, Dereymaeker G, Reynders P, et al. The management of chronic Achilles tendon ruptures: gastrocnemius turn down flap with or without flexor hallucis longus transfer. Foot Ankle Surg 2003;9:151–6.

50. Perez Teuffer A. Traumatic rupture of the Achilles tendon. Reconstruction by transplant and graft using the lateral peroneus brevis. Orthop Clin North Am 1974;5:89–93.

51. Mann RA, Holmes GB Jr, Seale KS, et al. Chronic rupture of the Achilles tendon: a new technique of repair. J Bone Joint Surg Am 1991;73:214–9.
52. Wapner KL, Pavlock GS, Hecht PJ, et al. Repair of chronic Achilles tendon rupture with flexor hallucis longus tendon transfer. Foot Ankle 1993;14:443–9.
53. Maffulli N, Leadbetter WB. Free gracilis tendon graft in neglected tears of the Achilles tendon. Clin J Sport Med 2005;15:56–61.
54. Bugg El Jr, Boyd BM. Repair of neglected rupture or laceration of the Achilles tendon. Clin Orthop Relat Res 1968;56:73–5.

Index

Note: Page numbers of article titles are in **boldface.**

A

Abductor hallucis longus tendon transfer, for hallux varus, 88, 91
Achilles tendon
    calcific insertional tendinopathy of, **113–123, 125–132**
    lengthening of, after partial foot amputations, 103–104
    rupture of, repair of
        complications of, 168–172
        failure of, **153–162**
        tendon and bone allograft combination for, **125–137**
    surgery on, complications of, 168–172
    tenectomy of, after partial foot amputations, 104–105
    tenotomy of, after partial foot amputations, 104–105
Adhesions, prevention of, 10
Advanced glycation end products, 5, 166
Allografts, bone, combined with tendon tissue, for Achilles tendon rupture, **125–137**
Amputation
    for clawfoot, 56
    partial foot, soft tissue balancing after, **99–111**
Ankle, arthrodesis of, after partial foot amputation, 103
Arthrodesis
    naviculocuneiform, for posterior tibial tendon dysfunction, 28
    of ankle, after partial foot amputation, 103
    subtalar, after partial foot amputation, 103
    tarsometatarsal, for posterior tibial tendon dysfunction, 22, 27–28
Arthrography, for complex deformities of digits and metatarsophalangeal joints, 75

B

Biomechanics, of tendon transfers, **1–13**
Blix curve, 4
Blood supply, for tendons, 2–3
Bone, tendon fixation to, 11
Bone grafts, combined with tendon tissue, for Achilles tendon rupture, **125–137**
Bowstringing effect, after posterior tibial tendon transfer, 38
Button technique, for tendon fixation, 11

C

Calcaneus, osteotomy of
    for calcific insertional Achilles tendinopathy, 117, 121
    for posterior tibial tendon dysfunction, 23–26
Calcific insertional Achilles tendinopathy, **113–123, 125–137**

Clin Podiatr Med Surg 33 (2016) 177–184
http://dx.doi.org/10.1016/S0891-8422(15)00106-8
0891-8422/16/$ – see front matter © 2016 Elsevier Inc. All rights reserved.

Cast, for posterior tibial tendon transfer, 36
Cavus foot
    correction of, with soft tissue release, **139–152**
    Jones tendon transfer for, **55–62**
Charcot-Marie-Tooth disease
    clawfoot in, Jones tendon transfer for, 56
    Hibbs tenosuspension for, **63–69**
Chopart amputation, soft tissue balancing after, 102–103
Cigarette smoking, tendon surgery healing and, 164–165
Clawfoot, Jones tendon transfer for, **55–62**
Clawing
    of hallux, Jones tendon transfer for, **55–62**
    of toes, after posterior tibial tendon transfer, 37
Clubfoot, tibialis anterior tendon transfer for, **41–53**
Cobb procedure, for posterior tibial tendon dysfunction, **21–28**
Collagen, in tendon composition, 2–5
Complex regional pain syndrome, after Achilles tendon surgery, 170
Contracture
    equinovarus, soft tissue release for, **139–152**
    of toes, Hibbs tenosuspension for, **63–69**
Corticosteroids, for complex deformities of digits and metatarsophalangeal joints, 75
Cuboid, tibialis anterior tendon transfer to, 46–47
Cuneiform, tibialis anterior tendon transfer to, 46–47

D

Debridement, of failed Achilles tendon repair, 155–156
Deep venous thrombosis, after Achilles tendon surgery, 170–171
Diabetes mellitus
    collagen structure in, 5
    tendon surgery complications in, 165–167
Donor tendons, selection of, 8–9
Dorsiflexory wedge osteotomy, with Jones tendon transfer, 60
Dropfoot
    posterior tibial tendon transfer for, **29–40**
    tibialis anterior tendon transfer for, **41–53**

E

Endotenon, 2
Epitenon, 2
Equinovarus deformity
    rigid, **139–152**
        biomechanics of, 140–141
        case reports for, 145–152
        causes of, 140
        clinical presentation of, 141
        evaluation of, 141–142
        surgical techniques for, 142–145
    tibialis anterior tendon transfer for, **41–53**

Equinus deformity, Hibbs tenosuspension for, **63–69**
Expendable tendon donor, 9
Extensor digitorum brevis tendon transfer
for complex deformities of digits and metatarsophalangeal joints, 80
in Hibbs tenosuspension, 66–67
Extensor digitorum longus tendon transfer
for complex deformities of digits and metatarsophalangeal joints, 80
in Hibbs tenosuspension, **63–69**
Extensor hallucis brevis tenodesis, for hallux varus, 95–96
Extensor hallucis longus tendon transfer
for clawfoot, 55–62
for hallux varus, 88–90
Extensor tendons, tenodesis of, after partial foot amputations, 108

F

Fascicles, structure of, 2
Femoral artery, occlusion of, equinovarus deformity in, 145–147
Fibrils, in tendon composition, 2
First dorsal interosseous tendon transfer, for hallux varus, 91
Fixation techniques, 10–11
Flatfoot
after posterior tibial tendon transfer, 37–38
in posterior tibial tendon dysfunction
flexor digitorum longus tendon transfer for, **15–20**
tibialis anterior tendon transfer for, **21–28**
Flexor digitorum longus muscle, contracture of, in equinovarus deformity, 143
Flexor digitorum longus tendon transfer
for calcific insertional Achilles tendinopathy, 118–120, **125–132**
for complex deformities of digits and metatarsophalangeal joints, 75–80
for failed Achilles tendon repair, 157–158
for posterior tibial tendon dysfunction, **15–20**
Flexor hallucis longus muscle, contracture of, in equinovarus deformity, 143
Flexor hallucis longus tendon
bone graft combined with, for Achilles tendon rupture, **125–137**
imbalance of, Jones tendon transfer for, 55–62
Flexor tendons, tenodesis of, after partial foot amputations, 108

G

Gastrocnemius-soleus complex, procedures on
after partial foot amputation, 103–106
for calcific insertional Achilles tendinopathy, 116
"Gift box" technique, for Achilles tendon repair, 171
Girdlestone procedure, 75
Golgi tendon organs, 3
Grafts
for Achilles tendon repair, 171
skin, for failed Achilles tendon repair, 158–160

H

Hallux, claw, Jones tendon transfer for, **55–62**
Hallux malleus, Jones tendon transfer for, **55–62**
Hallux varus, **85–98**
    causes of, 85, 87
    tendon transfer for
        indications for, 85
        procedure options for, 88–96
Haloperidol, adverse reaction to, equinovarus deformity in, 147–149
Hamilton sign, 74
Healing, of tendon transfers, **163–175**
Hibbs tenosuspension, **63–69**

I

Immobilization, after tendon transfer, 11
Infection, of repaired Achilles tendon rupture, **153–162**
Interference screw, for tibialis anterior tendon transfer, 46–47
Interphalangeal joint, fusion of, in Jones tendon transfer, 55–62
Inversion, of foot, loss of, in posterior tibial tendon transfer, 37

J

Jones tendon transfer, **55–62**

K

Kidner technique, modified, for posterior tibial tendon dysfunction, **15–20**

L

Lachmann stress test, 74
Lateral column lengthening, for posterior tibial tendon dysfunction, 24, 26–27
Leg, thrombosis of, equinovarus deformity in, 149–152
Length-tension curve, 4
Lisfranc amputation, soft tissue balancing after, 102
Loop techniques, for tendon fixation, 11

M

Magnetic resonance imaging
    for calcific insertional Achilles tendinopathy, 115–116
    for complex deformities of digits and metatarsophalangeal joints, 75
Medial displacement calcaneal osteotomy, for posterior tibial tendon dysfunction, 23–26
Metatarsophalangeal joint
    complex deformities of, **71–84**
        causes of, 72–73
        complications of, 81
        conservative treatment of, 74–75
        diagnosis of, 74–75

rehabilitation in, 80
    surgical treatment of, 75–82
    deformity of, Jones tendon transfer for, 55–62
Midsubstance, of tendon, 2–3
Muscle(s)
    strength of, 6–7, 43
    synergistic transfers of, 9
    tendon transfer effects on, 6–7
Musculotendinous junction, 2–3

N

Navicular, flexor digitorum longus tendon attachment to, 15–20
Naviculocuneiform arthrodesis, for posterior tibial tendon dysfunction, 28
Nerve conduction studies, for posterior tibial tendon transfer, 32
Neurologic disorders
    clawfoot in, Jones tendon transfer for, 56
    equinovarus contracture in, **139–152**
    posterior tibial tendon transfer for, 31
    tendon dysfunction in, 3
Nicotine use, tendon surgery healing and, 164–165
Nonsteroidal anti-inflammatory drugs, for complex deformities of digits and
    metatarsophalangeal joints, 75

O

Osteotomy, calcaneal
    for calcific insertional Achilles tendinopathy, 117, 121
    for posterior tibial tendon dysfunction, 23–26

P

Paratenon, 2, 10
Partial foot amputations, soft tissue balancing after, **99–111**
Peroneal muscles, evaluation of, for posterior tibial tendon transfer, 31–32
Peroneal tendons
    surgery on, complications of, 167–168
    transfer of, after partial foot amputation, 107–108
Peroneus brevis tendon
    bone graft combined with, for Achilles tendon rupture, **125–137**
    contracture of, in equinovarus deformity, 143–144
    for failed Achilles tendon repair, 157–158
Peroneus longus tendon
    contracture of, in equinovarus deformity, 143–144
    for failed Achilles tendon repair, 157–158
    imbalance of, Jones tendon transfer for, 55–62
Peroneus tertius tendon transfer, 66
Physical therapy, 6
    after tendon transfer, 11–12
    for posterior tibial tendon transfer, 36
Pie-crusting technique, for skin plasty, for equinovarus deformity, 144–145

Plantar fascial release, in equinovarus deformity, 144
Plantar plate, dysfunction of, complex deformities in, 72–75
Ponseti technique, for tibialis anterior tendon transfer, 42
Posterior capsular contracture, in equinovarus deformity, 143
Posterior tibial tendon
    anatomy of, 30–31
    biomechanics of, 30–31
    contracture of, in equinovarus deformity, 143
    harvesting of, 33–34
    strength of, 31
Posterior tibial tendon dysfunction
    flexor digitorum longus tendon transfer for, **15–20**
    stages of, 15–16, 21–28
    tibialis anterior tendon transfer for, **21–28**
Posterior tibial tendon transfer, **29–40**
    complications of, 37–38
    history of, 32
    indications for, 31
    postoperative care for, 36–37
    preoperative considerations for, 31–32
    technique for, 32–35
    theory of, 32
Predislocation syndrome, complex deformities in, 72, 74–75
Pulvertaft weave, 11

R

Radiography
    for calcific insertional Achilles tendinopathy, 115
    for complex deformities of digits and metatarsophalangeal joints, 74-75
    for Jones tendon transfer, 58
Range of motion, tendon transfers and, 7–8, 11–12
Rehabilitation, after tendon transfer, 11–12
Reverse abductor hallucis transfer, for hallux varus, 92–95

S

Sarcomere length, 4
Silfverskiold test, 142
Skin graft, for failed Achilles tendon repair, 158–160
Skin plasty, for equinovarus deformity, 144–145
Smoking, tendon surgery healing and, 164–165
Soft tissue balancing, after partial foot amputations, **99–111**
Soft tissue bed, for tendon transfer, 8
Soft tissue release, for cavus foot, **139–152**
Spastic equinovarus deformity, **139–152**
Split extensor hallucis longus tendon transfer, for hallux varus, 91–92
Split tibialis anterior tendon transfer, **41–53**, 106–107
Spring ligament, reconstruction of, 22
Stiffness, after complex deformity correction, 81
Strapping, for complex deformities of digits and metatarsophalangeal joints, 75

Stretching, of tendons, 4
Stroke, equinovarus contracture in, **139–152**
Subtalar arthrodesis, after partial foot amputation, 103
Sural neuritis, after Achilles tendon surgery, 169–170
Sutures and suturing
    for Achilles tendon repair, 171
    for tendon transfer, 11
Synergy, in tendon transfer, 9

T

Tarsal tunnel decompression, for equinovarus deformity, 143
Tarsometatarsal arthrodesis, for posterior tibial tendon dysfunction, 22, 27–28
Tendinopathy, calcific insertional, of Achilles tendon, **113–123, 125–132**
Tendon(s)
    anatomy of, 1–2
    blood supply of, 2–3
    histology of, 2
    innervation of, 3
    strength of, 3–4
Tendon anchors, for tibialis anterior tendon transfer, 46–47
Tendon bone junction, 3
Tendon passers, for posterior tibial tendon transfer, 34–35
Tendon transfers
    after partial foot amputations, **99–111**
    biomechanics of, **1–13**
    complications of, **163–175**
    fixation for, 10–11
    for calcific insertional Achilles tendinopathy, **113–123, 125–132**
    for cavus foot, **55–62**
    for chronic Achilles tendon ruptures, **125–137**
    for clubfoot, **41–53**
    for complex digital deformities, **71–84**
    for digital contractures, **62–69**
    for dropfoot, **29–40**
    for equinovarus contracture, **139–152**
    for hallux malleus, **55–62**
    for hallux varus, **74–98**
    for infected Achilles tendon rupture, **153–162**
    for lesser metatarsophalangeal joint deformities, **71–84**
    for posterior tibial tendon dysfunction, **15–20**
    for posterior tibial tendon insufficiency, **21–28**
    healing of, **163–175**
    intraoperative considerations in, 9–10
    muscle balancing for, 6–7
    patient evaluation for, 4–7
    postoperative considerations in, 11–12
    principles of, **1–13,** 30
    rules of, 4–9
Tenosuspension, Jones, **55–62**
Thompson sign, 74, 126

Tibialis anterior tendon transfer, **41–53**
    complications of, 48–49
    for posterior tibial tendon dysfunction, **21–28**
    indications for, 42
    postoperative care for, 47
    rehabilitation for, 47–48
    results of, 48, 50–51
    subcutaneous, 50
    techniques for, 43–47
    transfer of, after partial foot amputation, 106–107
Tobacco use, tendon surgery healing and, 164–165
Toe(s)
    clawing of, after posterior tibial tendon transfer, 37
    complex deformities of, **71–84**
        causes of, 72–73
        complications of, 81
        conservative treatment of, 74–75
        diagnosis of, 74–75
        rehabilitation in, 80
        surgical treatment of, 75–82
Transmetatarsal amputation, soft tissue balancing after, 101–102
Transplantation, of tendon and bone allograft combination, for Achilles tendon rupture, **125–137**
Triple hemisection procedure, after partial foot amputations, 104
Tunnels, for tendon transfer, 10

U

Ulcers, Jones tendon transfer for, 57
Ultrasonography, for complex deformities of digits and metatarsophalangeal joints, 75

Y

Yu classification, for predislocation syndrome, 72

Moving?

Make sure your subscription moves with you!

To notify us of your new address, find your **Clinics Account Number** (located on your mailing label above your name), and contact customer service at:

Email: journalscustomerservice-usa@elsevier.com

800-654-2452 (subscribers in the U.S. & Canada)
314-447-8871 (subscribers outside of the U.S. & Canada)

Fax number: 314-447-8029

Elsevier Health Sciences Division
Subscription Customer Service
3251 Riverport Lane
Maryland Heights, MO 63043

Moving?

Make sure your subscription moves with you!

To notify us of your new address, find your Clinics Account Number (located on your mailing label above your name) and contact customer service at:

Email: journalscustomerservice-usa@elsevier.com

800-654-2452 (subscribers in the U.S. & Canada)
314-447-8871 (subscribers outside of the U.S. & Canada)

Fax number: 314-447-8029

Elsevier Health Sciences Division
Subscription Customer Service
3251 Riverport Lane
Maryland Heights, MO 63043

To ensure uninterrupted delivery of your subscription, please notify us at least 4 weeks in advance of move.